Heart Failure
Diagnosis and Management

Heart Failure
Diagnosis and Management

Edited by
Andrew L Clark MA MD MRCP
Senior Lecturer and Honorary Consultant Cardiologist
Academic Unit of Cardiology
Castle Hill Hospital
Hull
UK

John JV McMurray BSc MD FRCP FESC FACC
Professor of Cardiology
Clinical Research Initiative in Heart Failure
and Honoray Consultant Cardiologist, Western Infirmary
University of Glasgow
Glasgow
UK

MARTIN DUNITZ

© Martin Dunitz Ltd 2001

First published in the United Kingdom in 2001 by
Martin Dunitz Ltd
The Livery House
7–9 Pratt Street
London NW1 0AE
Tel: +44-(0)20-7482-2202
Fax: +44-(0)20-7267-0159
E-mail: info.dunitz@tandf.co.uk
Website: http://www.dunitz.co.uk

A CIP catalogue record for this book is available from the British Library

ISBN 1-85317-717-2

Distributed in the United States by:
Blackwell Science Inc.
Commerce Place, 350 Main Street
Malden MA 02148, USA
Tel: 1-800-215-1000

Distributed in Brazil by:
Ernesto Reichmann Distribuidora de Livros, Ltda
Rua Coronel Marques, 335–Tatuape 03440-000
Sao Paulo,
Brazil

Composition by Wearset, Boldon, Tyne & Wear
Printed and bound in Italy by Printer Trento

Contents

Contributors

Colin Berry MB ChB MRCP
MRC Clinical Training Fellow
Clinical Research Initiative in Heart Failure
University of Glasgow
Glasgow
UK

John Byrne MRCP
Specialist Registrar in Cardiology
Department of Cardiology
Western Infirmary of Glasgow
Glasgow
UK

Andrew L Clark MA MD MRCP
Senior Lecturer and Honorary Consultant Cardiologist
Academic Unit of Cardiology
Castle Hill Hospital
Hull
UK

Andrew P Davie
Specialist Registrar in Cardiology
Western Infirmary of Glasgow
Glasgow
UK

Samuel J McClure BSc MBChB MRCP
Specialist Registrar in Cardiology
Cardiology Department
Freeman Hospital
Newcastle upon Tyne
UK

John JV McMurray BSc MD FRCP FESC FACC
Professor of Cardiology
Clinical Research Initiative in Heart Failure
University of Glasgow and Honorary
Consultant Cardiologist, Western Infirmary
Glasgow
UK

David R Murdoch BMSc MBChB MRCP(UK)
Specialist Registrar in Cardiology and
Honorary Clinical Teacher
Department of Cardiology
Western Infirmary
Glasgow
UK

Neal Padmanabhan MA BM BCh MRCP(UK)
Lecturer in Clinical Medicine and Honorary
Specialist Registrar in Nephrology
Department of Medicine and Therapeutics
Western Infirmary of Glasgow
Glasgow
UK

Mark C Petrie
Specialist Registrar in Cardiology
Western Infirmary of Glasgow
Glasgow
UK

Simon Stewart BA BN Grad Dip Ad Ed PhD
NFESC
Ralph Reader Overseas Research Fellow
Clinical Research Initiative in Heart Failure
University of Glasgow
Glasgow
UK
and
Department of Cardiology
University of Adelaide
South Australia

Preface

Chronic heart failure is becoming a silent epidemic in industrialized nations. As more patients survive acute myocardial infarction due to advances in treatment, and as the population ages, chronic heart failure is becoming more common. It is all ready the commonest single cause for hospitalization. It has a mortality rate greater than that seen in most forms of neoplastic disease, and of the common chronic medical conditions carries the greatest burden of morbidity.

This combination of factors makes heart failure relatively easy to study. Recruitment to clinical trials is not difficult, and the hardest of end-points, death, is common. As a consequence there has been a large number of trials demonstrating mortality benefits for patients with heart failure with modern treatments.

The cornerstone of good management is an accurate diagnosis, and despite the incidence of heart failure, clinical diagnosis is notoriously unreliable. Even once the diagnosis has been made, treatment is often less than adequate; although much is known about the treatment of heart failure, too often patients are under-treated once the diagnosis is made. Part of the purpose of this book is to emphasize the importance of adequate treatment.

Non-drug measures can also help the lot of the patient with heart failure. These measures include manipulation of diet, exercise training regimens and various mechanical devices. An important recent development has been the appreciation of the role of specialist heart failure nurses. Specially trained nurses can reduce the morbidity of heart failure and possibly the mortality.

One of the successes of heart failure research has been the neurohormonal hypothesis in explaining both the progression of heart failure and the benefit of both angiotensin converting enzyme inhibitors and beta adrenoceptor antagonists. A range of new drugs is now in development targeted at various of the neurohormonal systems activated in response to heart failure.

Although the management of end-stage chronic heart failure is difficult, there is often something that can be done even for patients with the most intractable symptoms. New devices and surgical treatments are becoming available which are finding their place in heart failure therapy.

Heart failure is an exciting and fast moving area of cardiovascular medicine. It is so common that all doctors of whatever specialty will encounter it often. In this book, we aim to describe the rationale for modern heart failure management. Although heart failure is not curable, there is treatment available that greatly prolongs survival and improves quality of life. We owe it to our patients to make sure that they have access to the best available care.

Andrew L Clark
Hull, UK
John JV McMurray
Glasgow, UK

Chronic heart failure: the size of the problem

John JV McMurray

1

There is no doubt that heart failure is a major and growing public health problem in industrialized countries with ageing populations. Any attempt to describe the epidemiology of heart failure has, however, to take account of the difficulty in defining exactly what heart failure is. Although the focus of this chapter is the symptomatic syndrome it must be remembered that as many patients again have asymptomatic left ventricular systolic dysfunction, which might also be considered a form of 'heart failure'. Comprehensive reviews of the epidemiology and associated healthcare burden of heart failure have been published by Cowie et al,[1] McMurray et al[2] and McMurray and Stewart.[3] The full list of references for the studies cited in this chapter can be found in these articles.

Data relating to the aetiology, epidemiology and prognostic implications of heart failure are principally available from five types of study:

- Cross-sectional and longitudinal follow-up surveys of well-defined populations. These have almost exclusively focused on those individuals with clinical signs and symptoms indicative of chronic heart failure.
- Cross-sectional surveys of individuals who have been

medically treated for signs and symptoms of heart failures within a well-defined region.

- Echocardiographic surveys of individuals within a well-defined population to determine the presence of left ventricular systolic dysfunction.
- Nationwide studies of annual trends in heart failure-related hospitalization identified on the basis of diagnostic coding at discharge.
- Comprehensive clinical registries collected in conjunction with clinical trials. These include a large proportion of individuals who were identified on the basis of having both impaired left ventricular systolic dysfunction and signs and symptoms of heart failure.

Within the context of the specific limitations of the type of data available from these studies, the current understanding of the aetiology, epidemiology and prognostic implications of chronic heart failures are discussed here.

Epidemiology of heart failure

Prevalence

Table 1.1 summarizes the reported prevalence of heart failure according to whether this was estimated from a survey of individuals requiring medical treatment from a general practitioner or from population screening.

Despite the wide variation in the reported prevalence of heart failure (undoubtedly caused by differing research methods, in addition to inherent differences in the sociodemographic and risk factor profiles of study cohorts), overall, these data demonstrate that the prevalence of clinically overt heart failure increases markedly with age. These data also suggest that the prevalence of heart failure has increased over the past few decades.

Studies of patients visiting a general practitioner

Over the past 40 years in the UK there have been several large studies examining the number of patients being treated by a general practitioner for signs and symptoms of chronic heart failure. Only some of the more recent of these can be reviewed here. For example, Paramshwar et al[4] examined the clinical records of diuretic-treated patients in three general practices in northwest London in 1992 to identify possible cases of heart failure. From a total of 30 204 patients, a clinical diagnosis of heart failure was made in 117 cases (46 male and 71 female), giving an overall prevalence of 3.9 cases/1000. The prevalence of heart failure increased markedly with age—from a rate of 0.6 cases/1000 in those under 65 years to 28 cases/1000 in those aged over 65 years. Objective investigation of left ventricular function was, however, undertaken in less than one-third of these

Table 1.1
Reported prevalence of heart failure

Study	Location	Overall prevalence rate	Prevalence rate in older age groups
Surveys of treated patients			
RCGP (1985)	UK national data	3/1000	—
Gibson et al (1966)	Rural cohort, USA	9–10/1000	65/1000 (>65 yrs)
RCGP (1986)	UK national data	11/1000	—
Parameshwar et al (1992)	London, UK	4/1000	28/1000 (>65 yrs)
Rodeheffer (1993)	Rochester, UK	3/1000 (<75 yrs)	—
Mair et al (1994)	Liverpool, UK	15/1000	80/1000 (>65 yrs)
RCGP (1995)	UK national data	9/1000	74/1000 (65–74 yrs)
Clarke et al (1995)	Nottinghamshire, UK	8–16/1000	40–60/1000 (>70 yrs)
Population screening			
Droller and Pemberton (1953)	Sheffield, UK	—	30–50/1000 (>62 yrs)
Garrison et al (1966)	Georgia, USA	21/1000 (45–74 yrs)	35/1000 (65–74 yrs)
Framingham (1971)	Framingham, USA	3/1000 (<63 yrs)	23/1000 (60–79 yrs)
Landahl et al (1984)	Sweden (males only)	3/1000 (<75 yrs)	80–170/1000 (>67 yrs)
Eriksson et al (1989)	Gothenburg, Sweden	—	130/1000 (>67 yrs)
NHANES (1992)	USA national data	20/1000	80/1000 (>65 yrs)
Cardiovascular Health Study (1993)	USA national data	20/1000	80/1000 (>65 yrs)
RCGP (1995)	UK national data	9/1000 (25–74 yrs)	74/1000 (65–74 yrs)

See references 1–3 for full citations.

patients. Using similar methods, Mair et al[5] identified a total of 266 cases of heart failure from 17 400 patients within two general practices surveyed in Liverpool in 1994. The overall prevalence rate was 15 cases/1000 patients with 80 cases/1000 in those aged 65 years or over. More recently, Clarke et al[6] reported an even larger survey of heart failure based on similar methods and including analysis of prescription of loop diuretics for all residents of the English County of Nottinghamshire. They estimated that between 13 017 and 26 214 patients had been prescribed frusemide in this region of central England. Case note review of a random sample of those patients receiving such treatment found that 56% were being treated for heart failure. On this basis the investigators calculated an overall prevalence rate of 8–16 cases/1000. Once again, heart failure prevalence increased with advancing age, to 40–60 cases/1000 among those aged 70 years and over.

Population studies based on clinical criteria

There have now been many population studies of heart failure and only some can be reviewed here (see *Table 1.1*). At entry into the Framingham Study, 17 of 5209 persons (3 cases/1000) screened for heart failure on the basis of clinical criteria were thought to have heart failure; all were less than 63 years of age.[7] After 34 years of follow-up, prevalence rates increased as the cohort aged. The estimated prevalence of heart failure in the age groups 50–59, 60–69, 70–79 and 80 years and over was 8, 23, 49 and 91 cases/1000 persons, respectively.[8] The National Health and Nutrition Examination Survey (NHANES-1) screened 14 407 persons of both sexes, aged 25–47 years, between 1971 and 1975. This study mainly used self-reporting, and a clinical scoring system, with detailed evaluation of only 6913 subjects. The reported prevalence rate of heart failure in the US population was 20 cases/1000.[9] The study of men born in 1913 examined the prevalence of heart failure in a cohort of 855 Swedish

men at ages 50, 54, 57 and 67 years.[10] The prevalence rate of 'manifest' heart failure rose dramatically from 21 cases/1000 at age 50 years to 130 cases/1000 at age 67 years.

Prevalence of left ventricular systolic dysfunction

In only a few of the two types of prevalence study described above was objective evidence of cardiac dysfunction obtained. Consequently, it is unclear whether all patients really had heart failure and, if they did, what the cause of heart failure was. There have, however, been four recent estimates of the population prevalence of left ventricular systolic dysfunction, determined using echocardiography, conducted in Scotland,[11] the Netherlands, England and Finland. The Scottish study targeted a representative cohort of 2000 persons aged 25–74 years living north of the River Clyde in Glasgow. Of those selected, 1640 (82%) underwent a detailed assessment of their cardiovascular status. Left ventricular systolic dysfunction was defined as an echocardiographic left ventricular ejection fraction (LVEF) of ⩽30%. The overall prevalence of left ventricular systolic dysfunction using this criterion was 2.9%. Concurrent symptoms of heart failure were found in 1.5% of the cohort, whilst the remaining 1.4% were asymptomatic. Prevalence was greater in men and increased with age: in men aged 65–74 years it was

6.4% and in age-matched women 4.9%. The Rotterdam Study in the Netherlands, although examining individuals aged 55–74 years, reported similar findings. Overall, the prevalence of left ventricular systolic dysfunction, defined in this case as fractional shortening of ≤25%, was 5.5% in men and 2.2% in women.[12] The Helsinki Ageing Study[13] described the clinical and echocardiographic findings in 501 subjects (367 female) aged 75–86 years. The prevalence of heart failure, based on clinical criteria, was 8.2% overall (41 of 501) and 6.8%, 10% and 8.1% in those aged 75, 80 and 85, respectively. These individuals had a high prevalence of moderate or severe mitral or aortic valvular disease (51%), ischaemic heart disease (54%) and hypertension (54%). However, of the 41 subjects with 'heart failure', only 11 (27%) had significant left ventricular systolic dysfunction (diagnosed by the combined presence of fractional shortening of < 0.25 and left ventricular dilatation) and in 20 cases no echocardiographic abnormality was identified. Of the 460 without symptoms of heart failure, 43 (9%) also had left ventricular systolic dysfunction. The overall prevalence of left ventricular systolic dysfunction was therefore 10.8% (95% CI 8.2–13.8%). More recently, Morgan et al[14] studied 817 individuals aged 70–84 years selected from two general practices in Southampton, England. Left ventricular function was assessed qualitatively

as normal, mild, moderate or severe dysfunction. The overall prevalence of all grades of dysfunction was 7.5% (95% CI 5.8–9.5%). Prevalence of left ventricular dysfunction doubled between the ages of 70–74 years and > 80 years.

Preserved left ventricular systolic function

One of the most controversial issues about heart failure at present is the occurrence of the syndrome in patients with preserved left ventricular systolic function (and no other obvious cause, e.g. valvular disease). A full discussion of this topic is beyond the scope of this review. There are, however, two recent studies of this type of heart failure. The Olmsted County study, Minnesota, found that 43% of patients with chronic heart failure had LVEF of ≤50%.[15] Similarly, the Framingham investigators found that 49% of their cohort with heart failure had a LVEF of < 50%.[16] More recent work has suggested that, in the majority of patients presenting with possible heart failure with preserved left ventricular systolic function, there is an alternative explanation for their symptoms.[17]

Incidence

There is much less known about the incidence that the prevalence of heart failure. *Table 1.2* shows reported incidence rates from the largest population-based studies. The most detailed incidence data come from The Framingham Heart Study.[8] As in other population-based prevalence studies, heart failure was defined according to a clinical scoring system. The only 'cardiac' investigation was a chest X-ray. At 34 years' follow-up, the incidence of heart failure was approximately 2 new cases/1000 in persons aged 45–54 years, increasing to 40 new cases/1000 in men aged 85–94 years. Using similar criteria, the study of men born in 1913[10] reported incidence rates of 'manifest' heart failure of 1.5, 4.3 and 10.2 new cases/1000 in men aged 50–54, 55–60 and 61–67 years, respectively. The Rochester Epidemiology Project[18] also reported the incidence of heart failure in persons aged 0–74 years in a US population. The annual incidence was 1.1 new cases/1000. Once again the incidence was higher in men compared to women (1.57 versus 0.71 cases/1000, respectively). It also increased with age—the rate of new cases increasing from 0.76/1000 in men aged 45–49 to 1.6/1000 in men aged 65–69 years.

The most recent incidence study was reported by Cowie et al[19] From the Hillingdon district of London with a population of approximately 150 000. In a 15-month period, 122 patients were referred to a special heart failure clinic. This represented an annual referral rate of 6.5/1000 population. Using a broad definition of heart failure, only 29% of these patients were clearly diagnosed as having heart failure (annual incidence 1.85/1000 population).

Table 1.2
Reported incidence of heart failure

Study	Location	Incidence rate (whole population)	Incidence rate in older age groups
Eriksson et al (1989)	Sweden (men born in 1913)	—	10/1000 (61–67 yrs)
Remes et al (1992)	Eastern Finland	1–4/1000 (45–74 yrs)	8/1000 (>65 yrs)
Ho et al (1993)	Framingham, USA	2/1000	—
Rodeheffer et al (1993)	Rochester, USA	1/1000 (<75 yrs)	16/1000 (>65 yrs)
Cowie et al (1999)	London, UK	1/1000	12/1000 (>85 yrs)

See references 1–3 for full citations.

Heart failure admissions

A different type of epidemiological information comes from reports of heart failure-related hospital admissions on a country to country basis, although these also need to be interpreted with some caution, owing to their retrospective nature and variations in coding practices and changing admission thresholds over time. *Figure 1.1* shows the reported hospitalization rates from Scotland,[20] Spain, the USA, Sweden, New Zealand and the Netherlands for the period 1978–93. Hospitalization for heart failure appears to be a growing problem on a global scale. For example, studies undertaken in the UK suggest that in the early 1990s 0.2% of the population were hospitalized for heart failure per annum and that such admissions accounted for more than 5% of adult general medicine and geriatric hospital admissions— outnumbering those associated with acute myocardial infarction.[20] In the USA heart failure continues to be the most common cause of hospitalization in people over the age of 65 years.[21] Admissions for heart failure are frequently prolonged and, in many cases, followed by readmission within a short period of time. For example, in the UK the mean length of stay for a heart failure-related

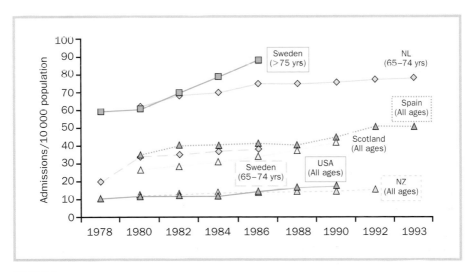

Figure 1.1
Comparison of heart failure admission rates per annum (recorded hospital admissions/10 000 population at risk) in Western developed countries, 1978–93. Adapted from data in reference 3.

admission in 1990 was 11.4 days on acute medical wards and 28.5 days on acute geriatric wards. Within the UK about one-third of patients are readmitted within 12 months of discharge, whilst the same proportion are reported to be readmitted within 6 months in the USA.[20,21] Such readmission rates are usually higher than the other major causes of hospitalization, including stroke, hip fracture and respiratory disease. Moreover, although there is evidence to suggest that an increasing number of heart failure patients are surviving a heart failure-related hospital admission, there is a parallel decrease in the number of patients who are discharged on an independent basis to their own homes. On a sex-specific basis, men tend to be younger than women when admitted for the first time with heart failure, but because of greater female longevity, the numbers of male and female admissions are roughly equal.

Cost of heart failure

In any healthcare system, hospital admissions represent a disproportionate component of total health care expenditure. Not surprisingly, considering the high rates of hospitalization for heart failure and the ongoing treatment and care it requires, the overall management of heart failure requires a significant amount of healthcare expenditure in industrialized nations. *Figure 1.2* shows that heart failure is reported to consume

between 1 and 2% of healthcare expenditure in a number of industrialized countries.[1] Moreover, considering the increasing rates of hospitalization, it is likely that these reported estimates fall short of the current burden of heart failure.

Aetiology of heart failure

In Western developed countries, coronary artery disease, either alone or in combination with hypertension, seems to be the commonest cause of heart failure. It is, however, very difficult to be certain of the primary aetiology of heart failure in a patient with multiple potential causes (e.g. coronary artery disease, hypertension, diabetes mellitus, atrial fibrillation, etc.). Furthermore, even the absence of overt hypertension in a patient presenting with heart failure does not rule out an important aetiological role in the past with normalization of blood pressure as the patient develops pump failure. Even in those with suspected coronary artery disease the diagnosis is not always correct and in the absence of coronary angiography must remain presumed rather than confirmed. In this context, even coronary angiography has its limitations in identifying atherosclerotic disease.

Common precursors of chronic heart failure are:

- Coronary artery disease (e.g. consequent upon acute myocardial infarction)

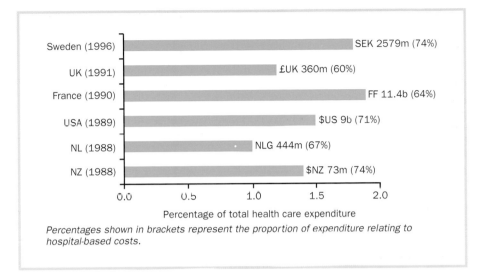

Percentages shown in brackets represent the proportion of expenditure relating to hospital-based costs.

Figure 1.2
The cost of chronic heart failure compared with the total health expenditure in the UK, Sweden, the Netherlands, France, New Zealand and the USA. The figures in brackets represent the component of hospital costs contributing to total expenditure quoted in the local currency and as a proportion of total healthcare expenditure for that country. Adapted from data in reference[3].

- Chronic hypertension
- Cardiomyopathy (e.g. dilated, hypertrophic, alcoholic and idiopathic)
- Valvular dysfunction (e.g. diseases of the aortic and mitral valve)
- Cardiac arrhythmias (e.g. heart block and atrial fibrillation)
- Pericardial disease (e.g. constrictive pericarditis)
- Infection (e.g. rheumatic fever, Chagas' disease, viral myocarditis and HIV)

The initial cohort of The Framingham Heart Study was monitored until 1965. Hypertension appeared to be the most common cause of heart failure, being identified as the primary cause in 30% of men and 20% of women and a co-factor in a further 33% and 25%, respectively. Moreover, electrocardiographic evidence of left ventricular hypertrophy in the presence of hypertension carried an approximately 15-fold increased risk of developing heart failure. In the subsequent years of follow-up, however, coronary heart disease became increasingly prevalent prior to the development of heart failure and, as the identified cause of new cases of heart failure, increased from 22% in the 1950s to almost 70% in the 1970s.[22] During this period, the relative contribution of hypertension and valvular heart disease declined dramatically. *Figure 1.3* is a summary of the changing association of coronary artery disease, hypertension, diabetes and valvular heart disease with the subsequent development of heart failure over the period 1950–87.[23] There was an approximately 5 and 30% decline in the prevalence per decade of hypertension during this period among men and women, respectively. The declining contribution of hypertension most probably reflects the introduction of antihypertensive therapy; the parallel decline in the prevalence of left ventricular hypertrophy supports this supposition. It is also probable that, during this same period, progressively greater accuracy in determining the presence of coronary heart disease contributed to its increasing importance in this regard.

As noted above, however, any interpretation of the Framingham data has to consider the fact that heart failure was identified on clinical criteria alone and undoubtedly included individuals without associated left ventricular systolic dysfunction. Conversely, the large-scale clinical trials

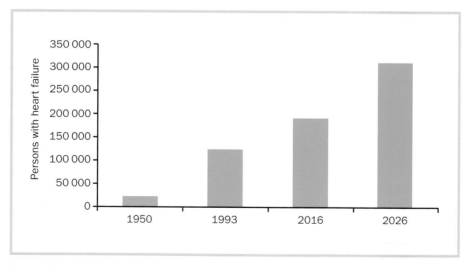

Figure 1.3
Changes in causal factors for heart failure in the Framingham Heart Study during the period 1950–87. Adapted from Levy et al.[22]

largely recruited patients who had reduced LVEF and applied an extensive list of exclusion criteria. *Table 1.3* is a summary of the most common attributed causes and factors associated with heart failure in a number of clinical trials and registries.[24–30] Coronary artery disease appears to be the most common underlying cause of heart failure, consistent with the more recent Framingham experience.

In the study of left ventricular function in North Glasgow,[11] 95% versus 71% of symptomatic and asymptomatic individuals with definite left ventricular systolic dysfunction had evidence of coronary artery disease ($p = 0.04$). Those individuals with

Table 1.3
Aetiology of heart failure in clinical trials and registers

	Clinical trials					Registers	
	SOLVD[24] (1991)	DIG study[26] (1997)	MERIT-HF[27] (1999)	ATLAS[28] (1999)	RALES[25] (1999)	SOLVD (1992)	SPICE[30] (1999)
Size of cohort	2569	6800	3991	3192	1663	6273	9580
Mean age	61	64	64	64	65	62	66
Male (%)	80	78	78	79	73	74	74
Aetiology of heart failure (%)							
Ischaemic	71	70	66	64	54	69	63
Non-ischaemic	—	29	34	35	46	31	—
Hypertensive	—	(9)	—	(20)	—	7	4
IDCM	18	(15)	—	(28)	—	13	17
Valvular	—	—	—	(6)	—	—	5
Other	—	6	—	—	—	11	—
Unknown	—	—	—	—	—	—	6
Comorbidity (%)							
Hypertension	42	—	44	46	—	43	27
Diabetes	26	—	25	29	—	23	—
Atrial fibrillation	10	—	17	—	—	14	—
Current angina	37	—	—	27	—	—	—
Respiratory disease	26	—	—	—	—	15	—

IDCM, idiopathic dilated cardiomyopathy

symptomatic heart failure were also more likely to have suffered a past myocardial infarction (50% versus 14%); $p = 0.01$) and concurrent angina (62% versus 43%; $p = 0.02$). Hypertension (80%) and valvular heart disease (25%) were also more prevalent in those individuals with both clinical and echocardiographically determined heart failure compared to the remainder of the cohort— including those with asymptomatic left ventricular dysfunction (67% and 0%, respectively).[11] One recent study, however, reports an unknown aetiology for heart failure in a disturbingly high proportion of cases.[19] Therefore, the aetiological importance of many of the associated causes of heart failure will depend on both the age cohorts examined and the type of criteria used to determine the presence of heart failure.

Prognosis

Heart failure, irrespective of whether it has been detected on the basis of being actively treated (e.g. during a hospital admission) or in otherwise asymptomatic individuals, is a lethal condition. There are some data to suggest that heart failure-related mortality is comparable to that of cancer. For example, in the original and subsequent Framingham cohort, the probability of someone with a heart failure diagnosis dying within 5 years was 62 and 75% in men and 38 and 42% in women, respectively.[31] In comparison, 5-year survival

for all cancers among men and women in the US during the same period was approximately 50%. The general applicability of these data is, however, limited by the few events recorded overall, the relative homogeneity of the Framingham population and the exclusion of older individuals. The Rochester Epidemiology Project has also described the prognosis in 107 patients presenting to associated hospitals with new-onset heart failure in 1981, and 141 patients presenting in 1991. The median follow-up in these cohorts was 1061 and 1233 days, respectively. The mean age of the 1981 patients was 75 years rising to 77 years in 1991. The 1-year and 5-year mortality was 28 and 66% in the 1981 cohort and 23 and 67% respectively, in the 1991 cohort.[32] In other words, although the same diagnostic criteria used in the Framingham study were used in the Rochester project, the prognosis was somewhat better in the latter.

The only other large, representative, epidemiological study reporting long-term outcome in patients with heart failure is the NHANES-1.[9] The initial programme evaluated 14 407 adults aged 25 and 74 years in the USA between 1971 and 1975. Follow-up studies were carried out in 1982–84 and again in 1986 (for those aged ≥55 years and alive during the 1982–84 review). The estimated 10-year mortality in subjects aged 25–74 years with self-reported heart failure was 42.8% (49.8% in men and 36% in women). Mortality in those aged 65–74 years was 65.4% (71.8 and 59.5% in men and women, respectively). These mortality rates are considerably lower than those observed in the Framingham study. The patients in NHANES-1 were non-institutionalized and their heart failure was self-reported. Follow-up was incomplete. NHANES-1 was also carried out in a more recent time period than Framingham when prognosis in heart failure patients may have improved. Framingham investigators in 1993 looked at patients developing heart failure in the period 1948–88 and the Rochester investigators in the period 1981–91. In both of these studies no temporal change in prognosis was identified.

It must be pointed out that all three of these studies describe a mixed population of patients, some of whom had systolic left ventricular dysfunction and others who did not. The true contribution of heart failure to overall mortality or coronary artery disease-related mortality is almost certainly underestimated. Although heart failure is highly prevalent among the elderly, it represents the terminal manifestation of a number of cardiovascular disease states and has been shown to be associated with extremely poor survival rates; official statistics continue to attribute only a small proportion of deaths to this syndrome. This reflects a common policy of coding the cause of death as the underlying aetiology (e.g. coronary artery disease rather than heart failure itself).

Future burden of heart failure

Despite an overall decline in age-adjusted mortality from coronary heart disease in developed countries overall, the number of patients with chronic coronary heart disease is increasing. This is principally the result of two separate trends. First, the proportion of elderly in the population is increasing rapidly and these subjects have the highest incidence of coronary heart disease and hypertension. Secondly, survival in those with coronary artery disease is improving. In particular, it has been shown that survival after acute myocardial infarction has increased markedly over the past decade, at least in part because of better medical treatment.[33] As coronary artery disease is the most powerful risk factor for heart failure (and its most important precursor) it is likely that the aforementioned trends will lead to an increase in its future prevalence. Chronic heart failure may, therefore, become a more common manifestation of chronic heart disease and contribute to many more deaths. Two formal projections of the future burden of heart failure have been undertaken in the Netherlands[34] and Australia.[35] For example, an analysis of demographic trends in the Netherlands has predicted that the prevalence of heart failure, due to coronary heart disease, will rise by approximately 70% during the period 1985–2010.

Summary

Heart failure represents a major and escalating public health problem. Despite some difficulties in reconciling information from the many types (and locations) of reported studies examining the burden and consequences of heart failure, the epidemiology, aetiology and prognosis of heart failure can be summarized as follows:

- The overall prevalence of clinically identified heart failure is estimated to be 3–20 cases/1000 population, but rises to >100 cases/1000 population in those aged ≥65 years.
- Prevalence of confirmed left ventricular systolic dysfunction also increases with age and is more common in men. However, these rates are far less than reported for the syndrome of heart failure.
- The overall, annual incidence of clinically overt heart failure in middle-aged men and women is approximately 0.1–0.2%. However, with each additional decade of life there is approximate doubling of this rate and the incidence of heart failure in those aged >85 years is approximately 2–3%.
- Although reported incidence rates are higher in men than in women, greater longevity in women tends to balance overall prevalence rates on a sex-specific basis.
- Heart-failure admission rates appear to be steadily increasing in all industrialized countries—especially among older individuals. Overall, annual admission rates for 1990 ranged from 10 to 40 admissions/10 000 population and increased to >75 admissions/10 000 population in those aged >65 years.
- The cost of managing heart failure in the early 1990s was estimated to be 1–2% of total healthcare expenditure. Because hospital care consumes a significant proportion of this expenditure, and rates of heart failure-related hospitalization have probably risen, this may be an underestimate of the current cost of heart failure.
- Heart failure is associated with an approximately 60% mortality rate within 5 years of diagnosis.
- The combination of increasing survival after acute myocardial infarction and increased longevity in Western developed nations is likely to lead to an increase in the overall prevalence of heart failure.

References

1. Cowie MR, Moster A, Wood DA et al. The epidemiology of heart failure. *Eur Heart J* 1997; **18**: 208–225.

2. McMurray JJ, Petrie MC, Murdoch DR, Davie AP. Clinical epidemiology of heart failure: public and private health burden. *Eur Heart J* 1998; **19**: 9–16.

3. McMurray JJV, Stewart S. Epidemiology, aetiology and prognosis and heart failure. *Heart* 2000; **83**: 596–602.

4. Parameshwar J, Shackell MM, Richardson A et al. Prevalence of heart failure in three general practices in north west London. *Br J Gen Pract* 1992; **42**: 287–289.

5. Mair FS, Crowley TS, Bundred PE. Prevalence, aetiology and management of heart failure in general practice. *Br J Gen Pract* 1996; **46**: 77–79

6. Clarke KW, Gray D, Hampton JR. How common is heart failure? Evidence from PACT (prescribing analysis and cost) data in Nottingham. *J Public Health Med* 1995; **17**: 459–464.

7. McKee PA, Castelli WP, McNamara PM et al. The natural history of congestive heart failure: the Framingham study. *N Engl J Med* 1971; **285**: 1441–1446.

8. Ho KK, Pinsky JL, Kannel WB, Levy D. The epidemiology of heart failure: The Framingham Study. *J Am Coll Cardiol* 1993; **22**: 6–13.

9. Schocken DD, Arrieta MI, Leaverton PE et al. Prevalence and mortality rate of congestive heart failure in the United States. *J Am Coll Cardiol* 1992; **20**: 301–306.

10. Eriksson H, Svardsudd K, Larsson B et al. Risk factors for heart failure in the general population: the study of men born in 1913. *Eur Heart J* 1989; **10**: 647–656.

11. McDonagh TA, Morrison CE, Lawrence A et al. Symptomatic and asymptomatic left-ventricular systolic dysfunction in an urban population. *Lancet* 1997; **350**: 829–833.

12. Mosterd A, de Bruijne MC, Hoes AW et al. Usefulness of echocardiography in detecting left ventricular dysfunction in population based studies (the Rotterdam study). *Am J Cardiol* 1997; **79**: 103–104.

13. Kupari M, Lindroos M, Iivanainen AM et al. Congestive Heart Failure in old age: prevalence, mechanisms and 4-year prognosis in the Helsinki ageing study. *J Intern Med* 1997; **241**: 387–394.

14. Morgan S, Smith H, Simpson I et al. Prevalence and clinical characteristics of left ventricular dysfunction among elderly patients in general practice setting: cross sectional survey. *BMJ* 1999; **318**: 368–372.

15. Senni M, Tribouilloy CM, Rodeheffer RJ. Congestive heart failure in the community: a study of all incident cases in Olmsted County, Minnesota, in 1991. *Circulation* 1998; **98**: 2282–2289.

16. Vasan RS, Larson MG, Benjamin EJ et al. Congestive heart failure in subjects with normal versus reduced left ventricular ejection fraction: prevalence and mortality in a population-based cohort. *J Am Coll Cardiol* 1999; **33**: 1948–1955.

17. Caruana L, Petrie MC, Davie AP, McMurray JJV. Do patients with suspected heart failure and preserved left ventricular systolic function suffer from 'diastolic heart failure' or from misdiagnosis? A prospective descriptive study. *Br Med J* 2000; **321**: 215–218.

18. Rodeheffer RJ, Jacobsen SJ, Gersh BJ et al. The incidence and prevalence of congestive heart failure in Rochester, Minnesota. *Mayo Clin Proc* 1993; **68**: 1143–1150.

19. Cowie MR, Wood DA, Coats AJ et al. Incidence and aetiology of heart failure; a population-based study. *Eur Heart J* 1999; **20**: 421–428.

20. McMurray J, McDonagh T, Morrison CE, Dargie HJ. Trends in hospitalization for heart

failure in Scotland 1980–1990. *Eur Heart J* 1993; **14:** 1158–1162.

21. Haldeman GA, Croft JB, Giles WH, Rashidee A. Hospitalization of patients with heart failure: national hospital discharge survey 1985–1995. *Am Heart J* 1999; **137:** 352–360.

22. Levy D, Larson MG, Vasan RS et al. The progression from hypertension to congestive heart failure. *JAMA* 1996; **275:** 1557–1562.

23. Kannel WB, Ho KK, Thom T. Changing epidemiological features of cardiac failure. *Eur Heart J* 1994; **72:** 3–9.

24. The SOLVD Investigators. Effect of enalapril on survival in patients with reduced left ventricular ejection fractions and congestive heart failure. *N Engl J Med* 1991; **325:** 293–302.

25. Pitt B, Zannad F, Remme WJ et al. The effect of spironolactone on morbidity and mortality in patients with severe heart failure. Randomized Aldactone Evaluation Study Investigators. *N Engl J Med* 1999; **341:** 709–717.

26. The Digitalis Investigation Group. The effect of digoxin on mortality and morbidity in patients with heart failure. *N Engl J Med* 1997; **336:** 525–533.

27. MERIT Investigators. Effect of metoprolol CR/XL in chronic heart failure: Metoprolol CR/XL Randomised Intervention Trial in Congestive Heart Failure (Merit-HF). *Lancet* 1999; **353:** 2001–2007.

28. Packer M, Poole-Wilson PA, Armstrong PW et al. Comparative effects of low and high doses of the angiotensin converting enzyme inhibitor, lisinopril, on morbidity and mortality in chronic heart failure. *Circulation* 1999; **100:** 2312–2318.

29. SOLVD Investigators. Natural history and patterns of current practice in heart failure. *J Am Coll Cardiol* 1993; **4A:** 14–19.

30. Bart BA, Ertl G, Held P et al. Contemporary management of patients with left ventricular systolic dysfunction. Results from the study of patients intolerant of converting enzyme inhibitors (SPICE) registry. *Eur Heart J* 1999; **20:** 1182–1190.

31. Ho KKL, Anderson KM, Karmel WB et al. Survival after the onset of congestive heart failure in the Framingham Heart Study subjects. *Circulation* 1993; **88:** 107–115.

32. Senni M, Tribouilloy CM, Rodeheffer RJ et al. Congestive heart failure in the community: trends in incidence and survival in a 10-year period. *Arch Intern Med* 1999; **159:** 29–34.

33. Rosamond WD, Chambless LE, Folsom AR et al. Trends in the incidence of myocardial infarction and in mortality due to coronary heart disease, 1987 to 1994. *N Engl J Med* 1998; **339:** 861–867.

34. Bonneux L, Barendregt JJ, Meeter K et al. Estimating clinical morbidity due to ischaemic heart disease and congestive heart failure: the future rise of heart failure. *Am J Public Health* 1994; **84:** 20–28.

35. Kelly DT. Our future society: a global challenge. *Circulation* 1997; **95:** 2459–2464.

Pathophysiology of chronic heart failure

Andrew L Clark

2

Introduction

Chronic stable heart failure is a clinical syndrome, and represents the end result of any process that results in sufficient loss of cardiac function. The process necessarily begins with damage to the heart, and the progress of heart failure is often described in terms of relentless downward spirals with the body's response to heart failure feeding back to cause further deterioration in cardiac function. Thus, a decline in cardiac output results in a fall in blood pressure; there is consequent sympathetic activation to maintain blood pressure, but this results in an increase in afterload with further decline in cardiac function (*Figure 2.1*).

The traditional model of heart failure describes the pathophysiology rather badly. Chronic heart failure is a multisystem disorder. Much evidence points to peripheral abnormalities as being at least as important as central haemodynamic function as determinants of exercise capacity, and perhaps of disease progression.

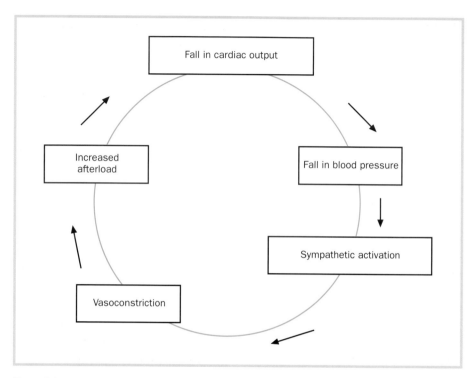

Figure 2.1
The vicious cycle of chronic heart failure

Symptomatology

Acute and chronic stable heart failure reflect two different underlying processes, although the originating event, defective cardiac function, is the same. Heart failure becomes chronic in part because the body's compensatory mechanisms have offset reduced cardiac function, and in part as a consequence of treatment (*Table 2.1*). From the patients'

perspective, chronic heart failure is a disease of exercise intolerance due usually to breathlessness or fatigue, or both. Perhaps surprisingly, the origin of the symptoms remains controversial.

By analogy with acute heart failure, breathlessness in chronic heart failure has traditionally been thought to arise from an acute rise in filling pressures on exercise with resultant 'wet lungs'. In this model, fatigue is

Table 2.1
Symptoms of chronic heart failure

> Oedema
> Exercise intolerance
>   Breathlessness
>   Fatigue
> Weight loss

ascribed to a failure of cardiac output to keep up with the metabolic demands of the exercising muscle. This supposes two distinct groups of patients being limited by distinct physiological problems: a breathless group, with wet lungs, and a fatigued group with impaired tissue perfusion. In fact, on formal exercise testing, it is difficult to distinguish between the two groups of patients,[1] suggesting that the two symptoms may represent a single underlying process.

Untreated chronic heart failure— 'dropsy'

Throughout human evolution, one of the major threats to life has been trauma. There has thus been an evolutionary premium on the development of biological systems to compensate for acute blood loss. These systems have centred around the response to an acute fall in blood pressure, drop in cardiac output and decrease in renal perfusion. The responses are corrective in that they cause salt and fluid retention, preserve blood flow to vital organs and stimulate thirst to replenish lost fluid volume. This is helpful when the fall in cardiac output has been due to assault by a sabre-toothed tiger, but may have adverse consequences when that fall is due to intrinsic cardiac disease. The pathophysiology of chronic heart failure reflects the evolutionarily programmed response of the organism to a fall in cardiac output, but in the absence of a fall in circulating volume.

The predominant finding in patients with untreated chronic heart failure is fluid retention and tissue oedema. Patients can be shown to have raised total body water and sodium,[2] although following treatment, fluid compartments return to normal.[3] Treated heart failure is frequently a disease of relapse and remission and the pattern of fluid retention and oedema is frequently repeated during the clinical course. The origin of salt and water retention is a decrease in renal perfusion (see *Figure 2.2*).

This physiological response is a reflection of the evolutionary imperative to retain fluid in response to trauma. The decreased renal perfusion causes excessive stimulation of the macula densa leading to increased renin secretion. In turn, the increased renin leads to the generation of angiotensin II and aldosterone. Angiotensin is a potent vasoconstrictor, and the resultant vasoconstriction causes increased peripheral resistance, and thus increased blood pressure. The increase in aldosterone secretion results in

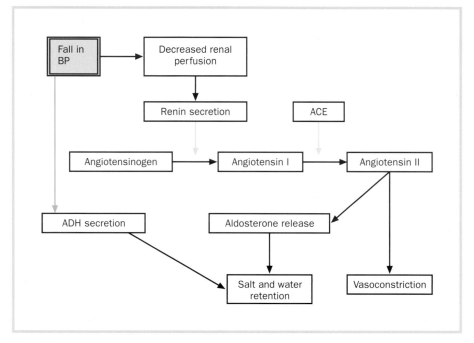

Figure 2.2
Origins of salt and water retention in chronic heart failure. The initiating event is seen to be a fall in blood pressure resulting in stimulation of antidiuretic hormone and the renin–angiotensin system. The net result is increased salt and water retention by the kidney. The mechanism by which ADH secretion is increased is not yet clear, nor is its relative importance

salt and water retention through its action at the distal tubule. In addition, antidiuretic hormone is secreted, causing increased water reabsorption from the collecting ducts in the kidney.

Exercise testing

It is difficult to assess subjective symptoms. Researchers have concentrated on the objective assessment of exercise responses using incremental exercise testing, often with metabolic gas exchange measurements. Using this type of approach, we can derive reasonably objective variables that describe exercise capacity. Peak oxygen consumption ($\dot{V}O_2$) is used as the indicator of exercise capacity, and progressively declines as heart failure progresses. The slope of the relationship between ventilation and carbon dioxide production ($\dot{V}E/\dot{V}CO_2$ slope) is taken as an index of the ventilatory response to exercise; the greater the ventilatory response to given carbon dioxide production (and the steeper the $\dot{V}E/\dot{V}CO_2$ slope), the greater the ventilatory response to exercise.

This approach suits the clinical scientist, producing objective and reproducible data.[4,5] It is, of course, a poor reflection of what troubles patients with chronic heart failure, who rarely meet with treadmills in daily life.[6] A variety of other tests has been developed, notably the 6-minute walk test. These have the merit of more accurately reflecting daily activities than maximal tests, but there are little available data relating these sorts of exercise tests to pathophysiology.

There are difficulties in using exercise testing to tease out the pathophysiology of heart failure. The normal response to exercise is relatively linear, at least at submaximal levels of exercise. For example, cardiac output, heart rate and ventilation all increase as a function of exercise load. Inevitably, at peak exercise, all these variables will correlate with each other. This should not be taken as evidence that one of these variables is the determinant of peak $\dot{V}O_2$.

A further difficulty is the amorphous nature of the heart failure syndrome itself. There are abnormalities in most of the body systems examined, and these abnormalities also progress as the disease progresses. Again inevitably, all these potential abnormalities will correlate between themselves, potentially suggesting causative relationships where none are truly present. Data relating to determinants of exercise capacity need to be interpreted with caution.

Pathophysiology

Abnormal cardiac function causes the heart failure syndrome, but is not closely connected with the pathophysiology of exercise limitation once the syndrome has developed. There are abnormalities of the circulation—central, peripheral and pulmonary—and abnormalities of pulmonary function. Recently, research interest has turned to abnormalities of the skeletal muscle, and the possible role abnormalities of physiological integration may play in the generation of symptoms.

The circulation

Central haemodynamics

One of the surprising features of heart failure physiology is that there appears to be little relationship between exercise capacity and indices of haemodynamic function. There is no relationship between peak $\dot{V}O_2$ and left ventricular filling pressures, left ventricular ejection fraction or resting cardiac output.[7,8] Acute improvements of haemodynamic function do not result in improved exercise capacity.[9–11] On the contrary, there is a gradual improvement after the administration of vasodilators over a period of weeks or months.[9,10]

A key observation is that submaximal cardiac output responses appear to be preserved in heart failure. At peak leg exercise, the addition of a further load in the form of arm exercise results in an increase in cardiac output and $\dot{V}O_2$ in heart failure patients in contrast with normal subjects.[12] It thus appears that, in normal subjects, exercise is limited by cardiac output, but in patients with chronic heart failure, something other than cardiac output is the limiting factor; the heart could work harder, but something else makes patients stop exercising.

An intriguing new approach has been to consider the possible role of the pericardium in heart failure. As the heart dilates, the pericardium can act to restrict cardiac filling. The dilated right heart may prevent the left ventricle from filling normally. When negative pressure is applied to the lower body, which should reduce venous return and thus cardiac filling pressures, a reduction in cardiac volumes is expected. In fact, in a proportion of heart failure patients, there is a paradoxical increase in left ventricular volume as right ventricular volume, and presumably

intrapericardial pressure, falls.[13] The importance of this diastolic ventricular interaction in heart failure physiology has not yet been established.

The peripheral circulation

The peripheral circulation adapts in heart failure to preserve perfusion to the brain and heart at the expense of the splanchnic circulation.[14] Blood flow to exercising muscle is also reduced,[15,16] with an impaired ability to vasodilate in response to exercise[17] and other stimuli.[18,19] This may be related to the development of abnormal skeletal muscle function (see below). There is near-maximal extraction of oxygen from the arterial blood, so that the femoral venous oxygen saturation can be extremely low.[20] This suggests that exercise may be limited by the capacity of the circulation to deliver oxygen to the muscles.

This may not be the whole story, however. Acute improvements in blood flow do not result in improved metabolism,[21] and some patients have normal leg blood flow, but abnormal muscle metabolism.[22]

The pulmonary circulation

There are weak correlations between peak $\dot{V}O_2$ and pulmonary vascular resistance, pressure and pulmonary capillary wedge pressure.[23,24] Some investigators have reported a relationship between right ventricular function and exercise capacity.[25] Others have not reproduced this finding, and in some patients with no functioning right ventricle at all, exercise capacity and the ventilatory response to exercise can be normal.[26]

Pulmonary function

Bronchoconstriction

Spirometric variables are abnormal in many patients with heart failure,[27] but certainly not invariably, particularly in non smokers.[28] Respiratory function tests in acute pulmonary oedema are consistent with airway obstruction.[29,30] There has been interest in the possibility that a rise in left atrial pressure results in congestion of the distal bronchial veins and hence bronchial wall oedema and bronchospasm,[31,32] but forced expiratory volume in one second (FEV_1) and forced vital capacity (FVC) decrease in parallel in treated chronic heart failure,[33] suggesting that obstructive lung pathology is unlikely to be a dominant problem. Whilst FEV_1 and FVC have been shown to be predictors of exercise capacity,[34] these are not necessarily variables specific for lung function. FEV_1, for example, is highly dependent on skeletal muscle function.

There is no evidence for increased bronchial hyper-responsiveness or exercise-induced bronchospasm.[35,36] Nitric oxide production, which is elevated in patients with inflammatory bronchoconstriction,[37,38] is not

increased in heart failure.[35] However, in some studies, nebulized bronchodilators given immediately before exercise result in an improvement in exercise capacity.[39] Some of these discrepancies may be explained by patient selection; patients with some airway disease due to smoking may respond to bronchodilators.

Pulmonary diffusion

Pulmonary diffusion capacity for carbon monoxide (DL_{CO}) is decreased in over 60% of heart failure patients,[40,41] even in many patients with normal lung volumes,[40] and after correction for lung volume.[42] Pulmonary diffusion can be broken into its components:

$$1/DL_{CO} = 1/D_M + 1/\theta V_C$$

where $1/DL_{CO}$ is total pulmonary diffusive resistance, $1/D_M$ is resistance at the alveolar capillary membrane, θ is the rate of reaction between carbon monoxide and haemoglobin, and V_C is the pulmonary capillary blood volume.[43]

DL_{CO} can thus be decreased where capillary blood volume is reduced, where the rate of reaction between haemoglobin and carbon monoxide is reduced, or where there is increased resistance at the alveolar capillary membrane. The impairment in pulmonary diffusion capacity appears to be due largely to increased resistance at the alveolar capillary membrane.[42,44] The resistance correlates with maximal exercise capacity and functional status, and inversely with pulmonary vascular resistance.

The origin of the decreased DLCO may lie with the observation of the resistance to pulmonary oedema despite high left heart filling pressures that some patients exhibit.[45] Repeated episodes of pulmonary oedema or chronically raised pressures may cause fixed structural abnormalities, which, whilst protecting against pulmonary oedema, result in a reduction of DLCO.

Respiratory sensation

A further possible contribution to breathlessness is stimulation of pulmonary J-receptors by accumulation of intrapulmonary fluid.[46] However, lignocaine administration results in no change in the sensation of dyspnoea, although suppressing the cough response to capsaicin.[47] Diamorphine administered before exercise resulted in an increase in exercise time, but no change in the ventilatory response to exercise or the sensation of breathlessness.[48] Abnormal activation of pulmonary receptors seems unlikely to be responsible for breathlessness.

Ventilation

One of the most consistent abnormalities of exercise in chronic heart failure is the increased ventilatory response. Ventilation is greater than normal at any given workload.[49-51] During the course of an incremental exercise test, minute ventilation increases as a linear function of carbon dioxide production. The overall ventilatory response can be summarized and quantified as the slope of this relationship—the $\dot{V}E/\dot{V}CO_2$ slope. The $\dot{V}E/\dot{V}CO_2$ slope is increased in heart failure, and correlates (inversely) with peak $\dot{V}O_2$—the worse the heart failure, the steeper the $\dot{V}E/\dot{V}CO_2$ slope.[52,53]

There has been much debate over the cause of the increased $\dot{V}E/\dot{V}CO_2$ slope. The relationship between ventilation and carbon dioxide production is described by the alveolar ventilation equation:

$$\dot{V}E/\dot{V}CO_2 = 863/(Pa,CO_2 \times (1 - VD/VT))$$

where Pa,CO_2 is the arterial carbon dioxide tension VD/VT is dead space described as a fraction of tidal volume and 863 is a constant to standardize all measurements to body temperature, pressure and saturation.

The $\dot{V}E/\dot{V}CO_2$ slope is abnormal from the onset of exercise,[54,55] suggesting that whatever is causing the increased slope is present at the outset, and is not the result of the early development of acidosis. Although it is not the same as 'breathlessness', it is certainly clinically relevant in defining a group of patients with poor prognosis.[56]

If carbon dioxide production is the

principle drive for ventilation, then in the face of near normal arterial P_{CO_2}, the cause of an increase in $\dot{V}E/\dot{V}CO_2$ must be an increase in $(1 - VD/VT)$, that is, an increase in dead space ventilation.

Anatomical dead space

The increase in dead space may arise from an altered ventilatory pattern. At any given minute ventilation, the respiratory rate is greater than normal in patients with chronic heart failure. The fixed anatomical dead space is thus ventilated more often, resulting in a greater proportion of the minute ventilation being dead space.[28,51] However, altering the ventilatory rate in normal subjects has no effect on the $\dot{V}E/\dot{V}CO_2$ slope.[57] This suggests that, at least in normal subjects, the lungs can compensate for changes in anatomical dead space. Nevertheless, low respiratory rates necessarily reduce VD/VT, and training at this ventilatory rate caused an increase in exercise capacity in heart failure patients.[58]

There may be a 'break point' in the plot of ventilation rate against tidal volume during exercise, so that the rate abruptly increases at the point when patients become breathless.[59] This may appear to explain an increase in dead space ventilation at peak exercise, but cannot explain the fact that the $\dot{V}E/\dot{V}CO_2$ is abnormal from the outset of exercise.[54,55] Other investigators have found that the slope relating tidal volume to frequency is the same

in both patients and controls.[60] Respiratory pattern is probably not an important determinant of ventilatory response to exercise.

Physiological dead space

This falls with exercise in heart failure,[61,62] but does not fall as far as in normal subjects.[28] Previous investigators have found from this evidence that dead space *per breath* is increased[61] and is the cause of the increased ventilatory response; an increase in dead space more generally has been widely accepted as the cause for the increased ventilatory response to exercise.[54,63,64] However, although VD/VT was higher at submaximal exertion in patients than in controls (although lower than at rest), absolute dead space ventilation was higher at peak exercise in controls than in patients, as was absolute dead space per breath (measured in litres, not as a fraction of tidal volume).[28]

Ventilation–perfusion matching

How might an increase in dead space arise? Abnormalities of the pulmonary circulation might account for this (*Figure 2.3*) with the right heart failing adequately to perfuse the lung apices. As we have seen above,[26] right heart function does not relate well to exercise capacity or ventilatory response.

Ventilation–perfusion ($\dot{V}/\dot{Q}$) mismatching

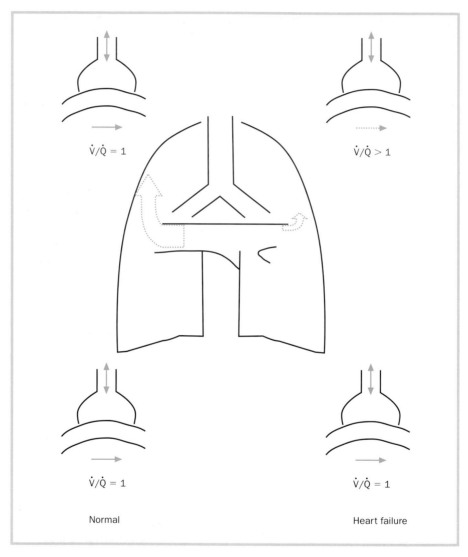

$\dot{V}/\dot{Q} = 1$

$\dot{V}/\dot{Q} > 1$

$\dot{V}/\dot{Q} = 1$

$\dot{V}/\dot{Q} = 1$

Normal

Heart failure

Figure 2.3
The possible origin of increased dead space. The right ventricle in the failing heart may lack the 'power' to perfuse the apices adequately. This will result in areas of lung being well ventilated but underperfused, thus causing increased dead space

improves during exercise in heart failure.[65] The reduction in mismatching correlates with exercise performance. The less $\dot{V}/\dot{Q}$ mismatching reduces with exercise, the shorter the exercise duration. However, it may simply be that $\dot{V}/\dot{Q}$ matching improves with increasing exercise load or duration and thus is a reflection of exercise done, not a determinant of exercise capacity.

A further observation is that perfusion to the lung apices appears to be increased in heart failure patients at rest,[66,67] and this does not change with exercise. This may imply that patients have better $\dot{V}/\dot{Q}$ matching than normal subjects at rest and at low levels of exercise; the apparent failure to reduce $\dot{V}/\dot{Q}$ mismatching as much as in normal subjects during exercise is explained as being due to having better matching at the start, rather than worse matching at the finish.

Pulmonary microcirculation

Experiments examining $\dot{V}/\dot{Q}$ matching on a large scale suggest that a primary lung abnormality is unlikely to be the cause for the increased $\dot{V}E/\dot{V}CO_2$ slope. There may be a microvascular problem in the lungs in heart failure, but experimental design has been too crude to detect this directly. Although systemic peripheral circulatory abnormalities have been described,[68–70] the pulmonary microcirculation is difficult to probe. Nitric oxide (NO) activity may be reduced in the

pulmonary circulation in heart failure,[71,72] although this is not universally reported.[73] There is evidence to suggest that, when NO is blocked, heterogeneity of resistance vessel behaviour can arise.[74] In addition, administration of nitric oxide during exercise results in a reduction in the $\dot{V}E/\dot{V}CO_2$ slope, although no change in VD/VT.[75]

Endothelin, a potent vasoconstrictor, is raised in heart failure; levels correlate with pulmonary vascular resistance,[76,77] and may be related to impaired endothelial responses to exercise. Hypoxia is a potential stimulus for vasoconstriction. Although systemic arterial hypoxaemia is not usually seen in chronic heart failure (see below), it may play a role in the lung; the low mixed venous oxygen saturation may cause vasoconstriction.[78] It is possible that some such mechanism may contribute to local disruption of $\dot{V}/\dot{Q}$ ratios, and an increase in dead space.

Ventilation and breathlessness

Despite the abnormalities of pulmonary function and ventilation, there is little objective evidence that these equate with breathlessness. At a given workload, patients have a greater minute ventilation than normal, but stop exercising at a much lower peak ventilation than normal.[28] There is little relation between exertional dyspnoea and measures of ventilatory function or demand.[79] A possible connection between ventilation and dyspnoea is that the work required for a given inspiratory volume is increased, thus altering the length–tension relationship in respiratory muscle, thus leading to dyspnoea.[80]

Blood gases

If some primary abnormality of pulmonary function were the driving force for the increased ventilatory response to exercise, one would expect some abnormality of blood gases to develop during exercise. In acute heart failure, blood gas abnormalities certainly occur with hypoxia[81] and less commonly carbon dioxide retention.[82]

There is a greater tendency to arterial desaturation in heart failure patients.[83] The increase in hypoxic episodes may represent the presence of periodic respiration, seen in some patients with heart failure.[84–86] The presence of oscillatory breathing during exercise is associated with a lower peak oxygen consumption.[87] There may be a subgroup of patients who do have desaturation as a clinically relevant problem. Increasing the fraction of inspired oxygen may result in an acute improvement in exercise capacity,[27] but this is not a consistent finding.[88]

Most studies of blood gases in exercise in *chronic* heart failure have shown no abnormality.[33,61,89] In those patients with an abnormality, some other pathology is present to account for it.[90] Indeed, it appears that hyperventilation occurs with respect to the

need for control of arterial blood gases during formal exercise testing.[28]

Arterial haemoglobin rises over the anaerobic threshold in chronic heart failure.[91] The arterial content of oxygen appears to be raised in chronic heart failure[92,93] with an increase in total body haemoglobin, which correlates inversely with cardiac function.[92] Arterial carbon dioxide content is also reduced.[94] These findings together suggest that, far from there being a primary lung problem in chronic heart failure inducing hyperventilation, the lungs cope well. There is likely to be a non-pulmonary component to the hyperpnoea of heart failure, and many of the apparent changes in pulmonary function may be secondary compensatory changes.

Chemoreceptors

Chemoreceptor activity is increased in chronic heart failure,[95] but the proportionate contribution to ventilation is the same in patients and controls (approximately 20%).[96] Patients with an enhanced chemoreflex drive have reduced exercise tolerance and an increased ventilatory response to exercise, as well as an increase in ventricular arrhythmias.[97] Suppression of the chemoreflex causes a reduction in the $\dot{V}E/\dot{V}CO_2$ slope.[98] The enhanced chemoreflex is also associated with baroreflex impairment and impaired autonomic control.[99]

An increased sensitivity to carbon dioxide

might explain the increased $\dot{V}E/\dot{V}CO_2$ slope in the presence of a reduction in arterial carbon dioxide tension. Sympathetic activation in normal subjects is associated with an increase in ventilation, possibly mediated via the chemoreceptors.[100] This could be relevant in chronic heart failure with its associated sympathetic activation.

Skeletal muscle

Patients with chronic heart failure have a skeletal muscle myopathy. Cardiac cachexia has been recognized for centuries,[101] but some degree of muscle wasting is common even in mild heart failure,[102] and is associated with a worsened prognosis.[103] The histology of skeletal muscle is abnormal with a relative reduction in oxidative type I fibres and a switch towards fast-twitch, glycolytic fibres (*Tables 2.2* and *2.3*).[104,105] Muscle biochemistry is abnormal, with a reduction in oxidative enzymes. There is early depletion of high-energy phosphate stores on exercise, and

intracellular acidosis.[106,107] Skeletal muscle has reduced strength,[108,109] and fatigues early.[110]

Similar changes affect respiratory muscle, with abnormalities in diaphragmatic histology,[111] reduced strength,[112] and endurance.[113] There is early respiratory muscle deoxygenation during exercise.[114] The work of breathing is increased in heart failure which may equate with the sensation of breathlessness.[115] Unloading of the work of breathing by using a helium–oxygen mixture results in an increase in exercise duration and improvement in the sensation of dyspnoea.[116] However, cardiac transplantation removes the sensation of dyspnoea whilst leaving the work of breathing unchanged,[117] suggesting that another factor is involved in the perception of breathlessness.

Sympathetic activation

Sympathetic activation is an important feature of chronic heart failure.[118] Its origin is not clear; traditionally, the baroreflex is thought to

Table 2.2
Skeletal muscle fibre types. In chronic heart failure, there is a shift towards type II fast-twitch glycolytic fibres

Fibre type	Colour	Function	Glycolytic capacity	Oxidative capacity
I	Red	Slow oxidative	Medium	High
IIa	Red	Fast oxidative	High	High
IIb	White	Fast glycolytic	High	Low

Table 2.3
Muscle abnormalities in chronic heart failure. Summary of information from a number of reports. Some aspects are more controversial than is perhaps indicated

Fibre type	I	↓
	IIa	↓
	IIb	↑
	IIc	↑
Glycolytic pathway		↔
Krebs' cycle		↓
Lipid oxidation		↓
Oxidative phosphorylation		↓
ATP/CrP		↓
Mitochondria		↓ volume
		↓ cristae
Capillary density/fibre		↓
/mm²		↓
		intracellular lipid, fibre atrophy

CrP, Creatine phosphate

mediate sympathetic activation, yet the baroreflex is down-regulated in chronic heart failure.[119,120] Ultrafiltration to remove over 3 l of body fluid, whilst resulting in a fall in blood pressure, results in suppression of the neurohormonal axis.[121] As mentioned above, enhanced chemoreceptor activity may be related to down-regulation of the baroreceptors.[103] Abnormal muscle signalling may also, in part, be responsible (see below).

Although sympathetic activation in the first instance appears to be beneficial in maintaining cardiac output, it is associated with a poor prognosis.[122] Adverse effects include an increase in peripheral resistance

and cardiac work, and may be related to the genesis of arrhythmias. Very high levels are associated with myocardial necrosis.[123] Recently, β-blockade has received a great deal of attention as a possible therapeutic intervention in heart failure.

Muscle signalling

Abnormal skeletal muscle seems to have an important role in heart failure. It is easy to envisage that the muscle will not perform well during exercise, resulting in fatigue. The abnormal respiratory muscle may contribute to the sensation of breathlessness. Skeletal muscle may make other important contributions to the pathophysiology of heart failure. There are muscle receptors responsive to work performed, and the response to stimulation of these receptors is termed the ergoreflex.[124] This reflex is enhanced in heart failure.[125] Simple experiments in normal subjects have shown that exercise with small muscle mass[126] or in ischaemic conditions[127] resulted in an increased ventilatory response to exercise. In addition, the enhanced ergoreflex was associated with an increase in sympathetic outflow.[125]

We can now hypothesize that the basic autonomic control systems are upset in chronic heart failure. A decrease in baroreflex activity is seen in chronic heart failure,[119,120] rather than the increase predicted from the usual model of heart failure. In contrast, the ergoreflexes and chemoreflexes, of only modest importance in normal subjects, become more active in patients with chronic heart failure. This model may explain some of the autonomic imbalance of heart failure (*Figure 2.4*).

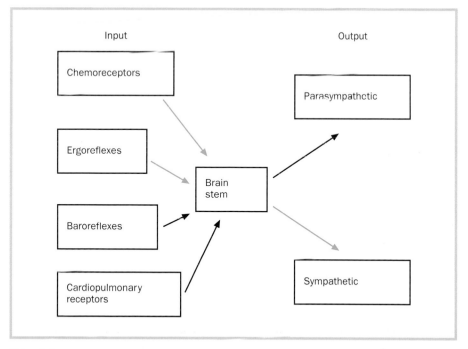

Figure 2.4a
Autonomic balance in health. Inputs lead predominantly to control by parasympathetic outflow

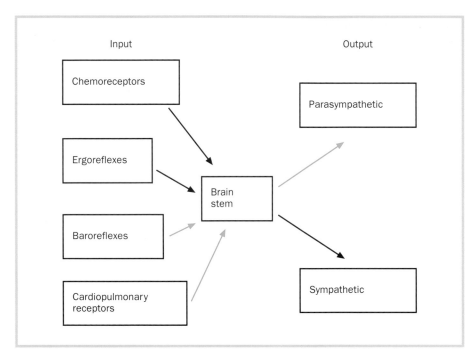

Figure 2.4b
In contrast, in chronic heart failure, the inputs to the cardiopulmonary centres in the brain stem are excitatory and result in an increase in sympathetic outflow

Immune activation and catabolic/anabolic imbalance

One of the striking abnormalities in chronic heart failure is the extent to which immune activation occurs. It is not obvious why this might be. Tumour necrosis factor α (TNFα) levels are elevated,[128,129] as are levels of its two receptors.[130] Pro-inflammatory cytokine levels are generally elevated.[131] Associated with this is evidence of a general imbalance between catabolic and anabolic hormonal factors. There is insulin resistance[132,133] and growth hormone resistance[134] with an elevation in both insulin and growth hormone, with reduced levels of insulin-like growth factor-I. Coupled to this is an increase in the catabolic steroid cortisol relative to the anabolic steroid dehydroepiandrosterone (DHEA).[130]

The consequences of immune activation

may include skeletal myopathy. Certainly, those patients with the most deranged catabolic/anabolic balance seem to be those most at risk of developing weight loss.[135] Weight loss has attracted interest recently, and seems to be important in predicting a group of patients with poor outcome.[103]

The origins of immune activation remain speculative. There is some preliminary evidence to support the hypothesis that exposure to bacterial endotoxin, perhaps as a result of bowel wall oedema, results in immune activation.[136] Whether this is the actual or only source of immune activation is not known. Certainly, immune activation represents a potential therapeutic target. A pilot study has shown promising results with etanercept.[137] Etanercept consists of two molecules of TNFα receptor connected to a portion of an immunoglobulin molecule. The molecule mops up circulating TNFα, making it biologically inert. A single infusion resulted in a reduction of TNFα bioactivity, an improvement in left ventricular ejection fraction and an improvement in quality of life. A larger-scale study, RENAISSANCE, will assess the effect of repeated dosing in larger numbers of patients.

Neurohormonal activation

Modern thinking on the progression of the heart failure syndrome has centred on the neurohormonal hypothesis.[138] Sympathetic

Table 2.4
Some of the neurohormones known to be activated in chronic heart failure

Neuropeptide Y
Vasoactive intestinal peptide
Calcitonin gene-related peptide
β-endorphin
Substance P
Prostaglandins
Adrenomedullin

(adrenergic) and renin–angiotensin system activation are two facets of this. Importantly, this has provided a framework for thinking about therapeutic strategies. Antagonizing these two systems has been a major step forward in heart failure management.

Many other hormonal systems are activated in heart failure (*Table 2.4*). For some of these, therapeutic modulation is being investigated, and is likely to become part of routine clinical practice.

Natriuretic peptides (ANP, BNP) are secreted by the atrial and ventricular myocardium in response to stretching. As their name implies, they induce diuresis. Basal levels are increased in heart failure. ANP and BNP are broken down to inactive metabolites by neutral endopeptidase (NEP), and NEP inhibitors are in development. The combined NEP/ACE inhibitor, omapatrilat, is in clinical trials.[139] A potential drawback is that NEP also catalyses the breakdown of potentially deleterious peptides, such as endothelin.

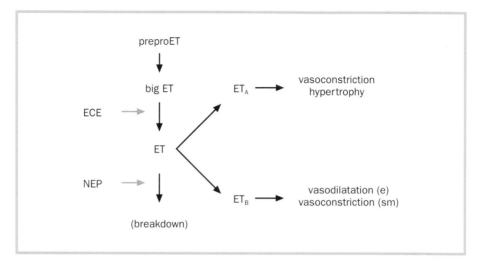

Figure 2.5
An outline of endothelin (ET) metabolism. There are, in fact, at least three endothelins, and more receptors. It may be that selective ET_A receptor blockade is more effective, leaving the potential vasodilatory ET_B receptors to remain stimulated. (e), endothelial cells; (sm), smooth muscle; ECE, endothelin converting enzyme; NEP, neutral endopeptidase. ET_A and ET_B are two subtypes of endothelin receptor

Endothelins are a group of very potent vasoconstrictors. They are increased in heart failure, particularly in those patients with pulmonary hypertension.[140] A diagram of endothelin metabolism is shown in *Figure 2.5*. Potential therapeutic targets include endothelin converting enzyme and endothelin receptors. Bosentan, which blocks both ET_A and ET_B receptors, has shown promising results in clinical trials.[141]

Vasopressin (arginine vasopressin, AVP or antidiuretic hormone, ADH) is elevated in some, but not all, patients with heart failure.

It acts via V_2 receptors in the collecting duct in the kidney to modulate the opening of the water channel, aquaporin 2.[142] Selective V_2 receptor antagonists are in development. These agents cause aquaresis with no salt loss, and may be of particular benefit to patients with hyponatraemia.

Integrated pathophysiology

This activation of immune systems and catabolic imbalance may be related to the skeletal myopathy, and in turn to the

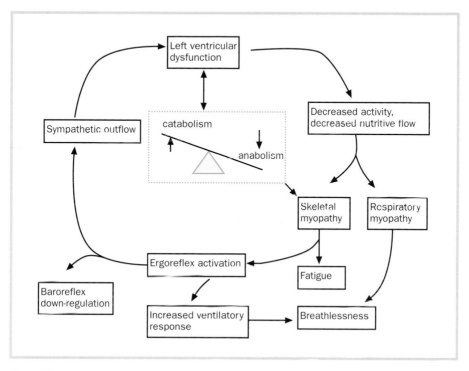

Figure 2.6
An alternative vicious cycle in chronic heart failure. There is a central role for skeletal muscle abnormalities in generating both symptoms and ergoreflex activation. Ergoreflex activation in turn drives sympathetic activation with its deleterious effects on the heart. Altered catabolic/anabolic balance has a crucial role in generating the muscle abnormalities, but its origins and relation to cardiac function remain unclear

development of symptoms. We can postulate a new vicious cycle of chronic heart failure with a central role for catabolic/anabolic imbalance (*Figure 2.6*). As a consequence of impaired cardiac function, skeletal myopathy develops, resulting in an exaggerated ergoreflex. In turn this leads to an increase in sympathetic activity and an enhanced ergoreflex contribution to the ventilatory response to exercise.

The sympathetic activation may be related to the subsequent down-regulation of the baroreceptors, perhaps allowing a greater relative contribution of the chemoreflexes to cardiovascular and pulmonary control than in normal subjects.

Conclusions

Chronic heart failure is a complex condition, and cannot be thought of simply as a failure of the circulation to meet the metabolic demands of the body. Practically no organ system is spared the effects of heart failure. This suggests many potential therapeutic interventions, such as treatment by exercise training, growth hormone or possibly immunotherapy during episodes of fluid retention. It may, too, assume greater importance that each individual patient be carefully characterized. In the future, therapeutic strategies may need to be tailored to the individual patient's needs, and may need to change frequently during the clinical course of the illness.

References

1. Clark AL, Sparrow JL, Coats AJS. Muscle fatigue and dyspnoea in chronic heart failure: two sides of the same coin? *Eur Heart J* 1995; **16:** 49–52.

2. Anand IA, Ferrari R, Kalra GS et al. Edema of cardiac origin: studies of body water and sodium, renal function, hemodynamic indexes, and plasma hormones in untreated congestive cardiac failure. *Circulation* 1989; **80:** 299–305.

3. Anand IS, Veall N, Kalra GS et al. Treatment of heart failure with diuretics: body compartments, renal function and plasma hormones. *Eur Heart J* 1989; **10:** 445–450.

4. Weber KT, Janicki JS. *Cardiopulmonary Exercise Testing.* WB Saunders, 1986: 154–155.

5. Hansen JE, Sue DY, Oren A, Wasserman K. Relation of oxygen uptake to work rate in normal men and men with circulatory disorders. *Am J Cardiol* 1987; **59:** 669–674.

6. Cowley AJ, Fullwood LJ, Muller AF et al. Exercise capability in heart failure: is cardiac output important after all? *Lancet* 1991; **337:** 771–773.

7. Fink LI, Wilson JR, Ferraro N. Exercise ventilation and pulmonary artery wedge pressure in chronic stable congestive heart failure. *Am J Cardiol* 1986; **57:** 249–253.

8. Franciosa JA, Park M, Levine TB. Lack of correlation between exercise capacity and indexes of resting left ventricular performance in heart failure. *Am J Cardiol* 1981; **47:** 33–39.

9. Massie BM, Kramer B, Haughom F. Acute and long-term effects of vasodilator therapy on resting and exercise hemodynamics and exercise tolerance. *Circulation* 1981; **64:** 1218–1226.

10. Drexler H, Banhardt U, Meinertz T et al. Contrasting peripheral short-term and long-term effects of converting enzyme inhibition in patients with congestive heart failure. A double-blind, placebo-controlled trial. *Circulation* 1989; **79:** 491–502.

11. Maskin CS, Forman R, Sonnenblick EH et al. Failure of dobutamine to increase exercise capacity despite haemodynamic improvement in severe chronic heart failure. *Am J Cardiol* 1983; **51:** 177–182.

12. Jondeau G, Katz SD, Zohman L et al. Active skeletal muscle mass and cardiopulmonary reserve: failure to attain peak aerobic capacity during maximal bicycle exercise in patients with severe congestive heart failure. *Circulation* 1992; **86:** 1351–1356.

13. Atherton JJ, Moore TD, Lele SS et al. Diastolic ventricular interaction in chronic heart failure. *Lancet* 1997; **349**: 1720–1724.

14. Zelis R, Flaim SF. Alterations in vasomotor tone in congestive heart failure. *Prog Cardiovasc Dis* 1982; **24**: 437–459.

15. Cowley AJ, Stainer K, Rowley JM, Hampton JR. Abnormalities of the peripheral circulation and respiratory function in patients with severe heart failure. *Br Heart J* 1986; **55**: 75–80.

16. Wilson JR, Martin JL, Schwartz D, Ferraro N. Exercise intolerance in patients with chronic heart failure: role of impaired nutritive flow to skeletal muscle. *Circulation* 1984; **69**: 1079–1087.

17. LeJemtel TH, Maskin CS, Lucido D, Chadwick BJ. Failure to augment maximal limb blood flow in response to one-leg versus two-leg exercise in patients with severe heart failure. *Circulation* 1986; **74**: 245–251.

18. Kubo SH, Rector TS, Bank AJ et al. Endothelium-dependent vasodilation is attenuated in patients with heart failure. *Circulation* 1991; **84**: 1589–1596.

19. Katz SD, Biasucci L, Sabba C et al. Impaired endothelium-mediated vasodilation in the peripheral vasculature in patients with congestive heart failure. *J Am Coll Cardiol* 1992; **19**: 918–925.

20. Clark AL, Volterrani M, Swan JW et al. Leg blood flow, metabolism and exercise capacity in chronic stable heart failure. *Int J Cardiol* 1996; **55**: 127–135.

21. Wilson JR, Martin JL, Ferraro N. Impaired skeletal muscle nutritive flow during exercise in patients with congestive heart failure: role of cardiac pump dysfunction as determined by the effect of dobutamine. *Am J Cardiol* 1984; **53**: 1308–1315.

22. Wilson JR, Mancini DM, Dunkman WB. Exertional fatigue due to skeletal muscle dysfunction in patients with heart failure. *Circulation* 1993; **87**: 470–475.

23. Franciosa JA, Baker BJ, Seth L. Pulmonary versus systemic hemodynamics in determining exercise capacity of patients with chronic left ventricular failure. *Am Heart J* 1985; **110**: 807–813.

24. Szlachcic J, Massie BM, Kramer BL et al. Correlates and prognostic implication of exercise capacity in chronic congestive heart failure. *Am J Cardiol* 1985, **55**: 1037–1042.

25. Baker BJ, Wilen MM, Boyd CM et al. Relation of right ventricular ejection fraction to exercise capacity in chronic left ventricular failure. *Am J Cardiol* 1984; **54**: 596–599.

26. Clark AL, Swan JW, Laney R et al. The role of right and left ventricular function in the ventilatory response to exercise in chronic heart failure. *Circulation* 1994; **89**: 2062–2069.

27. Moore DP, Weston AR, Hughes JMB et al. Effects of increased inspired oxygen concentrations on exercise performance in chronic heart failure. *Lancet* 1992; **339**: 850–853.

28. Clark AL, Volterrani M, Swan JW, Coats AJS. Increased ventilatory response to exercise in chronic heart failure: relation to pulmonary pathology. *Heart* 1997; **77**: 138–146.

29. Light RM, George RB. Serial pulmonary function in patients with acute heart failure. *Arch Intern Med* 1983; **143**: 429–433.

30. Peterman W, Barth J, Entzian P. Heart failure and airways obstruction. *Int J Cardiol* 1987; **17**: 207–209.

31. Cabanes LR, Weber SN, Matran R et al. Bronchial hyperresponsiveness to

methacholine in patients with impaired left ventricular function. *N Engl J Med* 1989; **320:** 1317–1322.

32. Cabanes L, Costes F, Weber S et al. Improvement in exercise performance by inhalation of methoxamine in patients with impaired left ventricular function. *N Engl J Med* 1992; **326:** 1661–1665.

33. Wasserman K, Zhang Y-Y, Gitt A et al. Lung function and exercise gas exchange in chronic heart failure. *Circulation* 1997; **96:** 2221–2227.

34. Kraemer MD, Kubo SH, Rector TS et al. Pulmonary and peripheral vascular factors are important determinants of peak exercise oxygen uptake in patients with heart failure. *J Am Coll Cardiol* 1993; **21:** 641–648.

35. Chua TP, Lalloo UG, Worsdell MY et al. Airway and cough responsiveness and exhaled nitric oxide in non-smoking patients with stable chronic heart failure. *Heart* 1996; **76:** 144–149.

36. Moore DP, Weston A, Hughes JMB et al. Bronchial hyperresponsiveness in heart failure. *N Engl J Med* 1993; **328:** 1424–1425.

37. Kharitonov SA, Yates D, Robbins RA et al. Increased nitric oxide in exhaled air of asthmatic patients. *Lancet* 1994; **343:** 133–135.

38. Kharitonov SA, Wells AU, O'Connor BJ et al. Elevated levels of exhaled nitric oxide in bronchiectasis. *Am J Repir Crit Care Med* 1995; **151:** 1889–1893.

39. Uren NG, Davies SW, Jordan SL, Lipkin DP. Inhaled bronchodilators increase maximum oxygen consumption in chronic left ventricular failure. *Eur J Cardiol* 1993; **14:** 744–750.

40. Wright RS, Levine MS, Bellamy PE et al. Ventilatory and diffusion abnormalities in potential heart transplant recipients. *Chest* 1990; **98:** 816–820.

41. Naum CC, Sciurba FC, Rogers RM. Pulmonary function abnormalities in chronic severe cardiomyopathy preceding cardiac transplantation. *Am Rev Respir Dis* 1992; **45:** 1334–1338.

42. Puri S, Baker BL, Dutka DP et al. Reduced alveolar-capillary membrane diffusing capacity in chronic heart failure. *Circulation* 1995; **91:** 2769–2774.

43. Roughton FJW, Forster FE. Relative importance of diffusion and chemical reaction rates in determining rate of exchange of gases in human lung, with special reference to true diffusing capacity of pulmonary membrane and volume of blood in the lung capillaries. *J Appl Physiol* 1957; **11:** 290–302.

44. Puri S, Baker BL, Oakley CM et al. Increased alveolar/capillary membrane resistance to gas transfer in patients with chronic heart failure. *Br Heart J* 1994; **72:** 140–144.

45. Wood P. An appreciation of mitral stenosis. *Br Med J* 1954; **1:** 1051–1063, 1113–1124.

46. Paintal AS. Mechanism of stimulation of type J pulmonary receptors. *J Physiol* 1969; **203:** 511–532.

47. Davies SW, Jordan SL, Newman S et al. Lignocaine aerosol anaesthesia and dyspnoea in chronic left heart failure. *Br Heart J* 1990; **64:** 59P (abstract).

48. Uren NG, Davies SW, Jordan SL, Lipkin DP. Increased exercise capacity after nebulised diamorphine in chronic heart failure. *Br Heart J* 1991; **66:** 112 (abstract).

49. Higginbotham MB, Morris KG, Conn EH et al. Determinants of variable exercise performance among patients with severe left

ventricular dysfunction. *Am J Cardiol* 1983; **51**: 52–60.

50. Rubin SA, Brown HV. Ventilation and gas exchange during exercise in severe chronic heart failure. *Am Rev Respir Dis* 1984; **129** (**Suppl**): S63–S64.

51. Weber KT, Kinasewitz GT, Janicki JS, Fishman AP. Oxygen utilisation and ventilation during exercise in patients with chronic cardiac failure. *Circulation* 1982; **65**: 1213–1223.

52. Buller NP, Poole-Wilson PA. Mechanism of the increased ventilatory response to exercise in patients with chronic heart failure. *Br Heart J* 1990; **63**: 281–283.

53. Davies SW, Emery TM, Watling MIL et al. A critical threshold of exercise capacity in the ventilatory response to exercise in heart failure. *Br Heart J* 1991; **65**: 179–183.

54. Metra M, Dei Cas L, Panina G, Visioli O. Exercise hyperventilation chronic congestive heart failure and its relation to functional capacity and hemodynamics. *Am J Cardiol* 1992; **70**: 622–628.

55. Milani RV, Mehra MR, Reddy TK et al. Ventilation/carbon dioxide production ratio in early exercise predicts poor functional capacity in congestive heart failure. *Heart* 1996; **76**: 393–396.

56. Chua TP, Ponikowski P, Harrington D et al. Clinical correlates and prognostic significance of the ventilatory response to exercise in chronic heart failure. *J Am Coll Cardiol* 1997; **29**: 1585–1590.

57. Clark AL, Coats AJS. Effects of induced changes in anatomical dead space ventilation on the relationship between ventilation and carbon dioxide production in normal man. *Eur J Clin Invest* 1993; **23**: 428–432.

58. Bernardi L, Spadacini G, Bellwon J et al. Effect of breathing rate on oxygen saturation and exercise performance in chronic heart failure. *Lancet* 1998; **351**: 1308–1311.

59. Yokoyama H, Sato H, Hori M et al. A characteristic change in ventilation mode during exertional dyspnea in patients with chronic heart failure. *Chest* 1994; **106**: 1007–1013.

60. Clark AL, Chua TP, Coats AJS. Anatomical dead space, ventilatory pattern, and exercise capacity in chronic heart failure. *Br Heart J* 1995; **74**: 377–380.

61. Sullivan MJ, Higginbotham MB, Cobb FR. Increased exercise ventilation in patients with chronic heart failure: intact ventilatory control despite haemodynamic and pulmonary abnormalities. *Circulation* 1988; **77**: 552–559.

62. Rajfer SA, Nemanich JW, Shurman AJ, Rossen JD. Metabolic responses to exercise in patients with heart failure. *Circulation* 1987; **76** (**Suppl VI**): VI46–VI53.

63. Myers J, Salleh A, Buchanan N et al. Ventilatory mechanisms of exercise intolerance in chronic heart failure. *Am Heart J* 1992; **124**: 710–719.

64. Wasserman K, Zhang Y-Y, Gitt A et al. Lung function and exercise gas exchange in chronic heart failure. *Circulation* 1997; **96**: 2221–2227.

65. Uren NG, Davies SW, Agnew JE et al. Reduction of mismatch of global ventilation and perfusion on exercise is related to exercise capacity in chronic heart failure. *Br Heart J* 1993; **70**: 241–246.

66. Mohensifar Z, Amin DK, Shah PK. Regional distribution of lung perfusion and ventilation in patients with chronic congestive heart failure and its relationship to cardiopulmonary

hemodynamics. *Am Heart J* 1989; **117**: 887–891.

67. Wada O, Asanoi H, Miyagi K et al. Importance of abnormal lung perfusion in excessive exercise ventilation in chronic heart failure. *Am Heart J* 1993; **125**: 790–798.

68. Kubo SH, Rector TS, Bank AJ et al. Endothelium-dependent vasodilation is attenuated in patients with heart failure. *Circulation* 1991; **84**: 1589–1596.

69. Katz SD, Biasucci L, Sabba C et al. Impaired endothelium-mediated vasodilatation in the peripheral vasculature of patients with congestive heart failure. *J Am Coll Cardiol* 1992; **19**: 918–925.

70. Katz SD, Schwartz M, Yuen J, Le Jemtel TH. Impaired acetylcholine-mediated vasodilation in patients with heart failure. *Circulation* 1993; **88**: 55–61.

71. Ontkean M, Gay R, Greenberg B. Diminished endothelium-derived relaxing factor in an experimental model of chronic heart failure. *Circ Res* 1991; **69**: 1088–1096.

72. Adachi H, Nguyen PH, Belardinelli R et al. Nitric oxide production during exercise in chronic heart failure. *Am Heart J* 1997; **133**: 196–202.

73. Habib F, Dutka D, Crossman D et al. Enhanced basal nitric oxide production in heart failure: another failed counter-regulatory vasodilator mechanism? *Lancet* 1994; **344**: 888–890.

74. Griffith TM, Edwards DH, Davies RL et al. EDRF coordinates the behaviour of vascular resistance vessels. *Nature* 1987; **329**: 442–444.

75. Bocchi EA, Auler JO, Guimarães GV et al. Nitric oxide inhalation reduces pulmonary tidal volume during exercise in severe chronic

heart failure. *Am Heart J* 1997; **134**: 737–744.

76. Cody RJ, Haas GJ, Binkely PF et al. Plasma endothelin correlates with the extent of pulmonary hypertension in patients with chronic congestive heart failure. *Circulation* 1992; **85**: 504–509.

77. Tsutamoto T, Wada A, Meada Y et al. Relation between endothelin-1 spillover in the lungs and pulmonary vascular resistance in patients with chronic heart failure. *J Am Coll Cardiol* 1994; **23**: 1427–1433.

78. Marshall C, Marshall B. Site and sensitivity of hypoxic pulmonary vasoconstriction. *J Appl Physiol* 1983; **55**: 711–716.

79. Russlel SD, McNeer FR, Higginbotham MB. Exertional dyspnea in heart failure: a symptom unrelated to pulmonary function at rest or during exercise. *Am Heart J* 1998; **135**: 398–405.

80. Campbell EM, Howell JBL. The sensation of breathlessness. *Br Med Bull* 1963; **19**: 36–40.

81. Fillmore SJ, Giumaraes AC, Scheidt SS, Kilip T. Blood gas changes and pulmonary hemodynamics following acute myocardial infarction. *Circulation* 1972; **45**: 583–591.

82. Aberman A, Fuplo M. The metabolic and respiratory acidosis of acute pulmonary edema. *Ann Intern Med* 1972; **76**: 173–184.

83. Munger MA, Stanek EJ, Nara AR et al. Arterial oxygen saturation in chronic congestive heart failure. *Am J Cardiol* 1994; **73**: 180–185.

84. Hanly P, Suberi N, Gray R. Pathogenesis of Cheyne–Stokes respiration on patients with congestive heart failure. Relationship to arterial P_{CO_2}. *Chest* 1993; **104**: 1079–1084.

85. Feld H, Priest S. A cyclic breathing pattern in patients with poor left ventricular function

and compensated heart failure: a mild form of Cheyne–Stokes respiration? *J Am Coll Cardiol* 1993; **21:** 971–974.

86. Mortara A, Sleight P, Pinna GD et al. Abnormal awake respiratory patterns are common in chronic heart failure and may prevent evaluation of autonomic tone by measures of heart rate variability. *Circulation* 1997; **96:** 246–252.

87. Kremser CB, O'Toole MF, Leff AR. Oscillatory hyperventilation in severe congestive heart failure secondary to idiopathic dilated cardiomyopathy or to ischemic cardiomyopathy. *J Am Coll Cardiol* 1987; **59:** 900–905.

88. Restrick LJ, Davies SW, Noone L, Wedzicha JA. Ambulatory oxygen in chronic heart failure. *Lancet* 1992; **334:** 1192–1193.

89. Rubin SA, Brown HV, Swan HJC. Arterial oxygenation and arterial oxygen transport in chronic myocardial failure at rest, during exercise and after hydralazine treatment. *Circulation* 1982; **66:** 143–148.

90. Clark AL, Coats AJS. Usefulness of arterial blood gas estimations during exercise in patients with chronic heart failure. *Br Heart J* 1994; **71:** 528–530.

91. Perego GB, Marenzi GC, Guazzi M et al. Contribution of pO_2, p50 and haemoglobin concentration to changes in artero-venous oxygen content during exercise in patients with heart failure. *J Appl Physiol* 1996; **80:** 623–631.

92. Herrlin B, Sylvén C. Increased arterial oxygen content – an important compensatory mechanism in chronic moderate heart failure. *Cardiovasc Res* 1991; **25:** 384–390.

93. Agostini PG, Wasserman K, Perego GB et al. Oxygen transport to muscle during exercise in chronic congestive heart failure secondary to idiopathic dilated cardiomyopathy. *Am J Cardiol* 1997; **79:** 1120–1124.

94. Hachamovitch R, Brown HV, Rubin SA. Respiratory and circulatory analysis of CO_2 output during exercise in chronic heart failure. *Circulation* 1991; **84:** 605–612.

95. Chua TP, Clark AL, Amadi A, Coats AJS. Relationship between chemosensitivity and the ventilatory response to exercise in chronic heart failure. *J Am Coll Cardiol* 1996; **27:** 650–657.

96. Chua TP, Ponikowski PP, Harrington D et al. Contribution of peripheral chemoreceptors to ventilation and the effects of their suppression on exercise tolerance in chronic heart failure. *Heart* 1996; **76:** 483–489.

97. Chua TP, Ponikowski PP, Webb-Peploe K et al. Clinical characteristics of chronic heart failure patients with an augmented peripheral chemoreflex. *Eur Heart J* 1997; **18:** 480–486.

98. Chua TP, Harrington D, Ponikowski P et al. Effects of dihydrocodeine on chemosensitivity and exercise tolerance in patients with chronic heart failure. *J Am Coll Cardiol* 1997; **29:** 147–152.

99. Ponikowski P, Chua TP, Piepoli M et al. Augmented peripheral chemosensitivity as a potential input to baroreflex impairment and autonomic imbalance in chronic heart failure. *Circulation* 1997; **96:** 2586–2594.

100. Clark AL, Galloway S, MacFarlane N et al. Catecholamines contribute to exertional dyspnoea and to the ventilatory response to exercise in normal humans. *Eur Heart J* 1997; **18:** 1829–1833.

101. Katz AM, Katz PB. Disease of the heart in works of Hippocrates. *Br Heart J* 1962; **24:** 257–264.

102. Mancini DM, Walter G, Reichnek N et al.

Contribution of skeletal muscle atrophy to exercise intolerance and altered muscle metabolism in heart failure. *Circulation* 1992; **85**: 1364–1373.

103. Anker S, Ponikowski P, Varney S et al. Wasting as an independent risk factor for mortality in chronic heart failure. Lancet 1997; **349**: 1050–1053.

104. Lipkin D, Jones D, Round J, Poole-Wilson P. Abnormalities of skeletal muscle in patients with chronic heart failure. *Int J Cardiol* 1988; **18**: 187–195.

105. Mancini DM, Coyle E, Coggan A et al. Contribution of intrinsic skeletal muscle changes to 31P NMR skeletal muscle abnormalities in patients with chronic heart failure. *Circulation* 1989; **80**: 1338–1346.

106. Massie BM, Conway M, Yonge R et al. Skeletal muscle metabolism in patients with congestive heart failure: relation to clinical severity and blood flow. *Circulation* 1987; **76**: 1009–1019.

107. Massie BM, Conway M, Yonge R et al. 31P nuclear magnetic resonance evidence of abnormal skeletal muscle metabolism in patients with congestive heart failure. *Am J Cardiol* 1987; **60**: 309–315.

108. Volterrani M, Clark AL, Ludman PF et al. Determinants of exercise capacity in chronic heart failure. *Eur Heart J* 1994; **15**: 801–809.

109. Buller NP, Jones D, Poole-Wilson PA. Direct measurements of skeletal muscle fatigue in patients with chronic heart failure. *Br Heart J* 1991; **65**: 20–24.

110. Minotti JR, Pillay P, Chang L et al. Neurophysiological assessment of skeletal muscle fatigue in patients with congestive heart failure. *Circulation* 1992; **86**: 903–908.

111. Lindsay DC, Lovegrove CA, Dunn MJ et al.

Histological abnormalities of muscle from limb, thorax and diaphragm in chronic heart failure. *Eur Heart J* 1996; **17**: 1239–1250.

112. Hammond MD, Bauer KA, Sharp JT, Rocha RD. Respiratory muscle strength in congestive heart failure. *Chest* 1990; **98**: 1091–1094.

113. Walsh JT, Andrews R, Johnson P et al. Inspiratory muscle endurance in patients with chronic heart failure. *Heart* 1996; **76**: 332–336.

114. Mancini DM, Ferraro N, Nazzaro D et al. Respiratory muscle deoxygenation during exercise in patients with heart failure demonstrated with near-infrared spectroscopy. *J Am Coll Cardiol* 1991; **18**: 492–498.

115. Mancini DM, Henson D, LaManca J, Levine S. Respiratory muscle function and dyspnea in patients with chronic congestive heart failure. *Circulation* 1992; **86**: 909–919.

116. Mancini D, Donchez L, Levine S. Acute unloading of the work of breathing extends exercise duration in patients with heart failure. *J Am Coll Cardiol* 1997; **29**: 590–596.

117. Mancini DM, LaManca J, Donchez L et al. The sensation of dyspnea during exercise is not determined by the work of breathing in patients with heart failure. *J Am Coll Cardiol* 1996; **28**: 391–395.

118. Francis GS, Goldsmith SR, Ziescke SM *et al.* Response of plasma norepinephrine and epinephrine to dynamic exercise in patients with congestive heart failure. *Am J Cardiol* 1982; **49**: 1152–1160.

119. Mohanty PK, Thames MD, Arrowood JA et al. Impairment of cardiopulmonary baroreflex in cardiac transplantation in humans. *Circulation* 1987; **75**: 914–921.

120. Ellenbogen KA, Mohanty PK, Szentpetery S, Thames MD. Arterial baroreflex abnormalities

in heart failure: reversal after orthotopic cardiac transplantation. *Circulation* 1989; **79**: 51–58.

121. Guazzi MD, Agostoni P, Perego B et al. Apparent paradox of neurohormonal axis inhibition after body fluid volume depletion in patients with chronic congestive heart failure and water retention. *Br Heart J* 1994; **72**: 534–539.

122. Cohn JN, Levine TB, Olivari MT et al. Plasma norepinephrine as a guide to prognosis in patients with chronic congestive heart failure. *N Engl J Med* 1984; **311**: 819–823.

123. Cruickshank JM, Degante JP, Kuurne T et al. Reduction of stress catecholamines induces cardiac necrosis by beta$_1$-selective blockade. *Lancet* 1987; **2**: 585–588.

124. Piepoli M, Clark AL, Coats AJS. Muscle metaboreceptors in the hemodynamic, autonomic and ventilatory responses to exercise in man. *Am J Physiol* 1995; **269** (*Heart Circ Physiol* **38**): H1428–H1436.

125. Piepoli M, Clark A, Volterrani M et al. Contribution of muscle afferents to the hemodynamic, autonomic and ventilatory responses to exercise in patients with chronic heart failure. *Circulation* 1996; **93**: 940–952.

126. Clark AL, Volterrani M, Piepoli M, Coats AJS. Factors which alter the relationship between ventilation and carbon dioxide production during exercise: implications for the understanding of the increased ventilatory response to exercise in chronic heart failure. *Eur J Appl Physiol* 1996; **73**: 144–148.

127. Clark AL, Piepoli M, Coats AJS. Skeletal muscle and the control of ventilation on exercise; evidence for metabolic receptors. *Eur J Clin Invest* 1995; **25**: 299–305.

128. McMurray J, Abdullah I, Dargie HJ, Shapiro D. Increased concentrations of tumour

necrosis factor in 'cachectic' patients with severe chronic heart failure. *Br Heart J* 1991; **66**: 356–358.

129. Levine B, Kalman J, Mayer L et al. Elevated circulating levels of tumour necrosis factor in severe chronic heart failure. *N Engl J Med* 1990; **323**: 236–241.

130. Anker SD, Clark AL, Kemp M et al. Tumour necrosis factor and steroid metabolism in chronic heart failure: possible relation to muscle wasting. *J Am Coll Cardiol* 1997; **30**: 997–1001.

131. Torre-Amione G, Kapadia S, Benedict C et al. Proinflammatory cytokine levels in patients with depressed ejection fraction: a report from the studies of left ventricular dysfunction (SOLVD). *J Am Coll Cardiol* 1996; **27**: 1201–1206.

132. Swan JW, Walton C, Godsland IF et al. Insulin resistance in chronic heart failure. *Eur Heart J* 1994; **15**: 1528–1532.

133. Swan JW, Anker SD, Walton C et al. Insulin resistance in chronic heart failure: relation to severity and etiology of heart failure. *J Am Coll Cardiol* 1997; **30**: 527–532.

134. Niebauer J, Pflaum C-D, Clark AL et al. Deficient insulin-like growth factor-I in chronic heart failure predicts altered body composition, anabolic deficiency, cytokine and neurohormonal activation. *J Am Coll Cardiol* 1998; **32**: 393–397.

135. Anker SD, Chua TP, Ponikowski P et al. Hormonal changes and catabolic/anabolic imbalance in chronic heart failure and their importance in cardiac cachexia. *Circulation* 1997; **96**: 526–534.

136. Anker SD, Egerer KR, Volk H D et al. Elevated soluble CD14 receptors and altered cytokines in chronic heart failure. *Am J Cardiol* 1997; **79**: 1426–1430.

137. Deswal A, Bozkurt B, Seta Y et al. Safety and efficacy of a soluble P75 tumor necrosis factor receptor (Enbrel, etanercept) in patients with advanced heart failure. *Circulation* 1999; **99**: 3224–3226.

138. Packer M. The neurohormonal hypothesis: a theory to explain the mechanism of disease progression in heart failure. *J Am Coll Cardiol* 1992; **20**: 248–254.

139. Witte K, Thachray S, Clark AL, Cleland JGF. Clinical trials update. *Eur J Heart Failure* 2000; **2**: 107–112.

140. Love MP, McMurray JJ. Endothelin in chronic heart failure: current position and future prospects. *Cardiovasc Res* 1996; **31**: 665–674.

141. Sütsch G, Kiowski W, Yan X-W et al. Short-term oral endothelin-receptor antagonist therapy in conventionally treated patients with symptomatic severe chronic heart failure. *Circulation* 1999; **98**: 2262–2268.

142. Schrier RW, Fassett RG, Ohara M, Martin PY. Vasopressin release, water channels, and vasopressin antagonism in cardiac failure, cirrhosis, and pregnancy. *Proc Assoc Am Physicians* 1998; **110**: 407–411.

Clinical diagnosis of heart failure

Andrew P Davie

3

The clinical diagnosis of heart failure is very difficult. Diagnosis requires a definition, and heart failure is very difficult to define, let alone diagnose; in fact, 'clinical diagnosis' of heart failure is almost a contradiction-in-terms, assuming that by clinical diagnosis we mean diagnosis based on the clinical interview (i.e. history and examination). Because the symptoms and signs of heart failure are so extremely non-specific, some other information is needed, and all the clinical picture can do is raise the suspicion that there may be heart failure. A clinical diagnosis of heart failure should always be substantiated by objective evidence of cardiac abnormality on further investigation,[1] and furthermore should preferably be confirmed by some degree of response to appropriate therapy.[2]

Even with (1) a working definition of heart failure, (2) an accepted method of confirmation of the diagnosis and (3) an appropriate regimen of treatment, novel concepts, such as diastolic heart failure, can emerge and call into question all three—definition, diagnosis and treatment. One way to minimize the confusion that this can engender is to ensure that terminology is always used rigorously. It is important to remember that heart failure is a syndrome and not a diagnosis.

Heart failure is most often (but not always) due to left ventricular systolic dysfunction, which is most often (but not always) due to ischaemic heart disease, which is most often (but not always) due to coronary artery disease, which is most often (but not always) due to coronary atherosclerosis. When we use the term 'heart failure' we tend to use it to encapsulate all these conditions, at least in our heads. Whilst we are most often right to do so, we must not forget the varied minority of conditions in which we are not.

Definition of heart failure

The simplest pathophysiological definition of heart failure was provided by Wood: 'a state in which the heart fails to maintain an adequate circulation for the needs of the body despite a satisfactory venous filling pressure.'[3] This was refined somewhat by Braunwald and Grossman in one of the most widely quoted definitions of heart failure: 'a state in which an abnormality of cardiac function is responsible for failure of the heart to pump blood at a rate commensurate with the requirements of the metabolising tissues or, to do so, only from an elevated filling pressure.'[4] A problem with such pathophysiological definitions is that many patients whom we would all recognize as having heart failure do not fit the definition. Many patients on treatment will have normal filling pressures and normal cardiac output at rest.

Others have emphasized the multisystem nature of the disorder, most notably Packer— 'A complex clinical syndrome characterised by abnormalities of left ventricular function and neurohormonal regulation which are accompanied by effort intolerance, fluid retention and reduced longevity'[5]—and Poole-Wilson—'A clinical syndrome caused by an abnormality of the heart and recognised by a characteristic pattern of haemodynamic, renal, neural and hormonal responses.'[6] Perhaps the most useful, certainly the most pragmatic, definition has been provided by the European Task Force: 'Symptoms of heart failure at rest or on effort, combined with objective evidence of cardiac dysfunction at rest, together with a response to treatment directed towards heart failure.'[2] All of these definitions emphasize to varying degrees the importance of objective evidence of cardiac (usually left ventricular) dysfunction (and latterly, the importance of a clinical response to treatment). The question arises to what extent that objective evidence can be provided by clinical assessment (without the help of the potentially compelling evidence gained from clinical intervention).

Symptoms of heart failure

The cardinal symptoms of heart failure are fluid retention (usually manifest as ankle swelling) and exercise intolerance, usually due to breathlessness and tiredness. Unfortunately

Table 3.1
Definition of sensitivity, specificity and positive and negative predictive values of a diagnosis of congestive heart failure (CHF)

	Test positive	Test negative
CHF present	True positive	False negative
CHF absent	False positive	True negative

Sensitivity = true positives/(true positives + false negatives) = proportion of patients with a positive test.
Specificity = true negatives/(true negatives + false positives) = proportion of non-CHF individuals with a negative result.
Positive predictive value = true positives/(true positives + false positives) = chance that a positive result is representative of CHF being present.
Negative predictive value = true negatives/(true negatives + false negatives) = chance that a negative result is representative of CHF being absent.
There is a trade-off between sensitivity and specificity. It is easy to design a sensitive test: 'does this person have a heart in their chest?' will be sensitive in that it detects all patients with heart failure (no false negatives), but hopelessly non-specific (everyone, whether CHF or not, tests positive).

these symptoms, even in combination, are very non-specific. Tiredness is probably the commonest and therefore least specific of all symptoms. The majority of patients presenting to their general practitioner complaining of tiredness ('I'm tired all the time, Doctor!') have little objective evidence of any pathophysiological abnormality,[7] let alone any cardiac abnormality. Nevertheless, tiredness is one of the most disabling symptoms of heart failure, and contributes to the extremely disabling nature of the disorder.[8] Symptoms of orthopnoea (breathlessness on lying flat) or paroxysmal nocturnal dyspnoea (waking with sudden-onset breathlessness during the night) might be expected to be more specific than breathlessness on exertion or breathlessness at rest, but are less common.

The symptoms of heart failure have been subjected to objective assessment, and sensitivity, specificity and positive and negative predictive values can be calculated for the purpose of objective comparison (see *Table 3.1* for definitions of these terms, *Table 3.2* and references 9–13 for results). Whilst orthopnoea and paroxysmal nocturnal dyspnoea can be seen to be much more specific than dyspnoea on exertion, they are much less sensitive. That is, whilst a clear majority (66–100%) of patients *with* confirmed heart failure *are* breathless on exertion (sensitivity), it is probably only a minority (15–52%) of similar patients *without* heart failure who do *not* have the same symptoms (specificity). In other words, many patients without heart failure are breathless on

Table 3.2
Sensitivity, specificity, positive and negative predictive value of symptoms in diagnosis of chronic heart failure

	Harlan (329 pts)	Chakko (52 pts)	Stevenson (50 pts)	Echeverria (50 pts)	Davie (259 pts)
DoE	66			97	100
	52			15	17
				63	18
				75	100
Orthopnoea	21	66	91	73	22
	81	47	100	40	74
		61	100	65	14
		37	64	50	83
PND	33			50	39
	76			45	80
				58	27
				38	87
AS	23	46	23	23	49
	80	73	100	70	47
		79	100	54	15
		37	18	38	83

DoE = dyspnoea on exertion; PND = paroxysmal nocturnal dyspnoea; AS = ankle swelling

exertion. Furthermore, whilst a probable majority (40–100%) of patients *without* confirmed heart failure do *not* have orthopnoea or paroxysmal nocturnal dyspnoea (specificity), it is probably only a minority (22–91%) of patients *with* confirmed heart failure who *do* have the same symptoms (sensitivity). It can also be seen that none of these symptoms achieves a significant positive predictive value, although the negative predictive value of breathlessness on exertion is very high. Only about one-third of patients (14–100%) with any of these symptoms are likely to turn out to have heart failure (positive predictive value), although the vast majority (75–100%) of patients without breathlessness on exertion will turn out not to have heart failure (negative predictive value). In short, these findings demonstrate that the presence of heart failure symptoms is *sensitive* but lacks specificity or predictive accuracy.

Table 3.3
Clinical signs of chronic heart failure

Signs of fluid overload	Ankle oedema
	Basal crackles
	Raised jugular venous pulsation
	Ascites
	Pleural effusion
Cardiac enlargement	Increased area of cardiac dullness
	Displaced apex beat
Cardiac strain	Tachycardia
	Third heart sound/gallop rhythm
	Decreased proportional pulse pressure
Miscellaneous	Pulsus alternans*
	Tricuspid regurgitation†
	Atrial fibrillation
	Dyskinetic apex

*See Figure 3.1; †see Figure 3.2

Signs of heart failure

The signs of heart failure might be expected to be more helpful in the clinical diagnosis of heart failure, more specific and, perhaps, more predictive of the presence of heart failure. After all, however expert the clinician's history-taking, he is still reliant upon the patient's subjective and untutored account. When it comes to clinical examination, the clinician's highly refined skills of objective assessment should surely come into play.

The signs of heart failure (*Table 3.3*) can be divided into three groups of signs representing different aspects of the condition:

- Signs of fluid retention (e.g. elevated jugular venous pulsation, pulmonary crackles and ankle oedema);

- Signs of cardiac enlargement (e.g. increased area of cardiac dullness to percussion and displaced apex beat);

- Signs of cardiac strain (e.g. tachycardia, decreased proportional pulse pressure and third heart sound).

These are mostly signs of decompensated heart failure, and whilst the diagnosis of decompensated heart failure may be relatively easy, decompensated heart failure is much less common than compensated heart failure. Furthermore, there is a limit to the extent to which any of these signs on their own has any particular sensitivity, specificity or predictive value for the diagnosis of heart failure (*Table 3.4* and references 9–16).

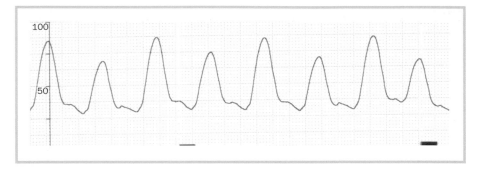

Figure 3.1
Pulsus alternans in a patient with severe chronic heart failure. Note the alternating high and low systolic pressure. (Scale in mmHg.)

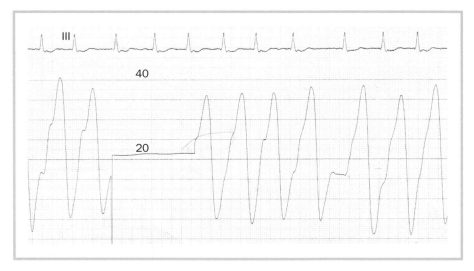

Figure 3.2
Pressure trace from the superior vena cava in a patient with severe heart failure and consequent tricuspid regurgitation. The rhythm is atrial fibrillation. Note the giant cV waves and mean pressure just above 20 mmHg.

Table 3.4
Sensitivity, specificity, positive and negative predictive value of signs in diagnosis of chronic heart failure

	Harlan (329 pts)	Heckerling (100 pts)	O'Neill (100 pts)	Chakko (52 pts)	Butman (52 pts)	Stevenson (50 pts)	Echeverria (50 pts)	Davie (259 pts)
↑P	7 / 99							22 / 92 / 33 / 86
↓PPP						91 / 8 / 91 / 87		0 / 100 / 84
↑JVP	10 / 97			70 / 79 / 85 / 62	57 / 93 / 95 / 47	58 / 100 / 100 / 28	47 / 65 / 67 / 45	17 / 98 / 64 / 86
↑DTP		94 / 67						
→AB			59 / 70 / 59 / 77				60 / 50 / 64 / 45	66 / 96 / 75 / 94
S3	31 / 95			73 / 42 / 66 / 85	68 / 73 / 86 / 48	98 / 14 / 88 / 50	63 / 55 / 68 / 50	24 / 99 / 77 / 87
Murmur								49 / 67 / 22 / 87
Crackles	13 / 91			66 / 84 / 87 / 61	24 / 100 / 100 / 35	19 / 100 / 100 / 17	70 / 35 / 62 / 44	29 / 77 / 19 / 85
Wheeze								12 / 82 / 11 / 83
Oedema	10 / 93			46 / 73 / 79 / 46		23 / 100 / 100 / 18	40 / 70 / 67 / 44	20 / 86 / 21 / 85

↑P = tachycardia; ↓PPP = decreased proportional pulse pressure; ↑JVP = jugular venous distension;
↑DTP = increased area of cardiac dullness to percussion; →AB = displaced apex beat; S3 = triple rhythm

Signs of fluid retention

Fluid retention in one form or another is regarded as almost pathognomic of heart failure. It is certainly part of the vicious cycle that characterizes decompensating heart failure (and is often the cause of the development of symptomatic heart failure in the first place). The definitions referred to earlier ('a state in which an abnormality of cardiac function is responsible for failure of the heart to pump blood at a rate commensurate with the requirements of the metabolising tissues or, to do so, only from an elevated filling pressure') make clear how fluid retention is an integral part of this vicious cycle. Failure of the heart to pump blood at a rate commensurate with the requirements of the kidneys results in reduced salt and water clearance and hence fluid retention. This initially compensates for the heart failure (allowing the heart to pump blood from an elevated filling pressure), but is ultimately deleterious, as the failing heart functions even less efficiently when subjected to prolonged elevation of filling pressures.

Despite the above considerations, signs of fluid retention are perhaps surprisingly non-specific. Ankle oedema (sensitivity 10–46%, specificity 70–100%, positive predictive value 21–100%, negative predictive value 18–85%) is more likely to be caused by chronic venous insufficiency than by congestive heart failure, especially in the middle-aged woman who complains also of tiredness and perhaps breathlessness on exertion. An elevated jugular venous pulsation (sensitivity 10–17%, specificity 65–100%, positive predictive value 64–100%, negative predictive value 28–86%) is quite a 'hard' sign, but is as likely to be caused by right heart failure secondary to pulmonary hypertension secondary to chronic pulmonary disease (cor pulmonale—not at all part of the spectrum of congestive heart failure) as it is by congestive heart failure. This is particularly so in the middle-aged or elderly chronic tobacco abuser who complains very justifiably of breathlessness on exertion. Pulmonary crackles (sensitivity 13–70%, specificity 35–100%, positive predictive value 19–100%, negative predictive value 17–85%) ought to be a very specific sign, but somehow they turn out not to be. This is perhaps because the crepitations of pulmonary alveolar oedema are so easily confused with those of chronic pulmonary disease or even those of stasis, especially if the patient does not clear his chest with a good cough. Ascites is an unusual (and late) sign of heart failure. It is difficult to elicit and needs to be approached with an open mind, as do other accumulations of fluid, such as pleural and pericardial effusions (similarly late signs of heart failure or worse).

Signs of cardiac enlargement

Signs of cardiac enlargement might be

expected to be more specific. After all, cardiac enlargement is surely a *sine qua non* of cardiac failure. That might be so if we accept the broadest possible definition of heart failure (expanded, for example, to include right heart failure), but not if we are interested in heart failure secondary to left ventricular systolic dysfunction. The different cardiac chambers have very different capacities to dilate. The left atrium can enlarge enormously (for example to 20 cm in diameter in severe chronic mitral valve disease). Similarly the right heart, especially the right atrium, can enlarge without imperilling cardiac function unduly. The left ventricle, on the other hand, only has to enlarge from around 5 cm to around 7 cm in diameter to be associated with severe left ventricular systolic dysfunction and severe chronic heart failure, and to around 9 cm to be barely compatible with life. It is only because *congestive* heart failure due to left ventricular systolic dysfunction is associated with *congestion*, and so with enlargement of the left atrium and right heart, that there is any useful association between cardiac size and heart failure at all. The usefulness of signs of cardiac enlargement is further compromised by the fact that they are rarely used in clinical practice and interobserver agreement is poor.[14,15,17] However, the evidence suggests that they may be useful clinical tools (increased area of cardiac dullness to percussion: sensitivity 94%, specificity 67%; displaced apex beat: sensitivity 59–66%,

specificity 50–96%, positive predictive value 59–75%, negative predictive value 45–94%).

Signs of cardiac strain

Signs of cardiac strain should clearly be very specific markers of heart failure. After all, they purport to detect the very thing we are looking for. Indeed, if the heart is failing, it must be doing so because it is under unacceptable strain (although, if it is under strain, that does not mean it is necessarily failing). However, the main problem with these signs is their subtlety, apart from tachycardia, which is all too easy to elicit (sensitivity 7–22%, specificity 92–99%, positive predictive value 33%, negative predictive value 86%). Decreased proportional pulse pressure, i.e. the proportion of systolic blood pressure over-and-above diastolic blood pressure (pulse pressure divided by systolic pressure; normal is above 30%), seems to be very difficult to elicit, as is a third heart sound.[18] One study claimed great sensitivity and predictive value for decreased proportional pulse pressure[11] (sensitivity 91%, specificity 8%, positive predictive value 91%, negative predictive value 87%), whereas another study did not find a single patient with heart failure who had a decreased proportional pulse pressure.[13] Eliciting a third heart sound is notoriously unreliable and subject to interobserver variability[18] (sensitivity 24–98%, specificity

14–99%, positive predictive value 66–88%, negative predictive value 48–87%).

Combinations of symptoms and/or signs

Clinical diagnosis is a process of pattern recognition. It is therefore somewhat unreasonable to suppose that any one symptom or sign would be at all specific, let alone sensitive, for the diagnosis of heart failure due to left ventricular systolic dysfunction. It is very much more complicated, and very difficult, to provide an objective assessment of the value of combinations of symptoms and signs. Certainly such combinations could be expected to be more specific and predictive, although less sensitive. Formal assessment of combinations has not often been attempted, but when most recently done, past history of myocardial infarction and displaced apex beat on examination emerged as the best single predictors of left ventricular systolic dysfunction, and a combination of these two was a very valuable combined predictor of left ventricular systolic dysfunction.[13] A medical history of myocardial infarction is in fact much more predictive of significant left ventricular systolic dysfunction than any conventional symptom, despite the fact that a minority of such patients have significant left ventricular systolic dysfunction.[19]

Scoring systems

It is a small step from looking at combinations of symptoms and signs to thinking of scoring systems for the diagnosis of heart failure.[20–25] There have been numerous attempts to devise such scoring systems, even equations for the calculation of left ventricular ejection fraction, but none of these has found common acceptance, perhaps because they are so much more complicated than simple investigations. In fact, most of them have included simple investigations, and cannot be held to be part of 'clinical' diagnosis. Scoring systems restricted to clinical information, readily volunteered symptoms and readily demonstrated signs have been mainly the preserve of epidemiologists. There have been three sets of clinical scoring systems in common use—the Framingham criteria,[26] the Duke criteria[9] and the Boston criteria,[22]—and these have mainly been used to define patients as having heart failure for epidemiological purposes. The fact that patients who fulfil these criteria are accepted as having heart failure, by definition, may be useful for epidemiological surveys, but it is hardly likely to be useful in clinical practice, given that we can all think of patients who would fulfil such criteria whom we would not regard as having heart failure.

A few examples

It may be useful to give a few examples of hypothetical patients, to give some idea of the thought processes involved in the clinical diagnosis of heart failure.

Mr A is 59 years old, a smoker, who had a myocardial infarction and coronary artery bypass grafting 10 years ago. He has recently noticed increasing breathlessness on exertion, which has responded somewhat to a diuretic. His examination is unremarkable. Despite this, the chances of Mr A having heart failure secondary to left ventricular systolic dysfunction are quite high, although the possibility or recurrent ischaemia or lung disease also deserves consideration. Investigation to confirm or deny this clinical impression is mandatory, considering the life enhancing treatments available.

Mrs B is 56 years old, 10 years postmenopausal and a smoker, who has had ankle swelling for years. More recently she has complained of weakness, tiredness and breathlessness. The ankle swelling has responded quite well to a diuretic, although the weakness and tiredness remain. Her examination is unremarkable apart from obesity and slight ankle swelling. The chances of Mrs B having heart failure secondary to left ventricular systolic dysfunction are slim. She merits further investigation, if only to help reassure her.

Miss C is 87 years old, and despite having kept very well all her long life, finds that she has slowed down recently. She is inclined to put her problems down to old age and wonders if she will be able to keep her second-floor flat much longer, given the number of times that she has to stop on the way up her 28 steps to pause for breath. Examination reveals a frail old lady, with obviously elevated jugular venous pulsation and an easily heard systolic murmur with some basal pulmonary crackles. Miss C may very well have heart failure, due to either left ventricular systolic dysfunction or valvular heart disease, and it is quite possible that she may be helped a great deal by appropriate medical or even surgical therapy.

Mr D is 69 years old, a heavy smoker who has worked both in the coalfields and in the shipyards. He complains of breathlessness on exertion. Thinking back, he finds that it has gone on for some years, but has become quite a problem recently. Examination reveals obesity and widespread pulmonary wheeze. He could have heart failure secondary to left ventricular systolic dysfunction, but is at least as likely to be developing angina of effort, or chronic lung disease.

Conclusions

The clinical diagnosis of heart failure is very difficult to make. It is important to have a high index of suspicion for the possibility of heart failure, but it is equally important that clinical suspicion be backed up by objective evidence of cardiac abnormality and preferably by a response to treatment as well. Only in this way will false-negative reassurance and false-positive diagnosis be avoided. Whilst the perils of inappropriate reassurance are obvious, false-positive diagnosis is also dangerous. Apart from the undesirability of providing patients with false information, the wrong diagnosis may lead to hazardous incorrect treatment and the omission of efficacious treatment. The clinical diagnosis of heart failure should not be attempted. Diagnosis of heart failure should always be backed up by appropriate use of tests. Like much else in clinical cardiology, this is a marked exception to the maxim that 90% of the diagnosis is in the history, 9% in the clinical examination and only 1% in the results of investigation.

References

1. Dargie HJ, McMurray JJV. Diagnosis and management of heart failure. *Br Med J* 1994; **308**: 321–328.

2. The Task Force on Heart Failure of the European Society of Cardiology. Guidelines for the diagnosis of heart failure. *Eur Heart J* 1995; **16**: 741–751.

3. Wood P. *Diseases of the Heart and Circulation.* London: Chapman and Hall, 1968.

4. Braunwald E, Grossman W. Clinical aspects of heart failure. In: Braunwald E (ed). *Heart Disease,* 4th edn. New York: WB Saunders, 1992: 444.

5. Packer M. Survival in patients with chronic heart failure and its potential modification by drug therapy. In: Cohn J (ed). *Drug Treatment of Heart Failure,* 2nd edn. Secaucus, NJ: ATC International, 1988: 273.

6. Poole-Wilson PA. Heart failure. *Med Int* 1985; **2**: 866–871.

7. Ridsdale L, Evans A, Jerrett W et al. Patients with fatigue in general practice: a prospective study. *Br Med J* 1993; **307**: 103–106.

8. Stewart AL, Greenfield S, Hays RD et al. Functional status and well-being of patients with chronic conditions. Results from the Medical Outcomes Study. *J Am Med Assoc* 1989; **262**: 907–913.

9. Harlan WR, Olberman A, Grimm R, Rosati RA. Chronic congestive heart failure in coronary artery disease: clinical criteria. *Ann Intern Med* 1977; **86**: 133–138.

10. Chakko S, Woska D, Martinez H et al. Clinical, radiographic, and hemodynamic correlations in chronic congestive heart failure: conflicting results may lead to inappropriate care. *Am J Med* 1991; **90**: 353–359.

11. Stevenson LW, Perloff JK. The limited reliability of physical signs for estimating hemodynamics in chronic heart failure. *J Am Med Assoc* 1989; **261**: 884–888.

12. Echeverria HH, Bilsker MS, Myerburg RJ, Kessler KM. Congestive heart failure: echocardiographic insights. *Am J Med* 1983; **75**: 750–755.

13. Davie AP, Francis CM, Caruana L et al. Assessing diagnosis in heart failure: which features are any use? *Q J Med* 1997; **90**: 335–339.

14. Heckerling PS, Wiener SL, Moses VK et al.

Accuracy of precordial percussion in detecting cardiomegaly. *Am J Med* 1991; **91**: 328–334.

15. O'Neill TW, Barry M, Smith M, Graham IM. Diagnostic value of the apex beat. *Lancet* 1989; **1**: 410–411.

16. Butman SM, Ewy GA, Standen JR et al. Bedside cardiovascular examination in patients with severe chronic heart failure: importance of rest or inducible jugular venous distension. *J Am Coll Cardiol* 1993; **22**: 968–974.

17. Dans AL, Bossone EF, Guyatt GH, Fallen EL. Evaluation of the reproducibility and accuracy of apex beat measurement in the detection of echocardiographic left ventricular dilatation. *Can J Cardiol* 1994; **11**: 493–497.

18. Ishmail AA, Wing S, Ferguson J et al. Interobserver agreement by auscultation in the presence of a third heart sound in patients with congestive heart failure. *Chest* 1987; **91**: 870–873.

19. McClure SJ, Caruana L, Davie AP et al. Cohort study of plasma natriuretic peptides for identifying left ventricular systolic dysfunction in primary care. *Br Med J* 1998; **317**: 516–519.

20. Marantz PR, Tobin JN, Wassertheil-Smoller S et al. The relationship between left ventricular systolic function and congestive heart failure diagnosed by clinical criteria. *Circulation* 1988; **77**: 607–612.

21. Remes J, Miettinen H, Reunanen A, Pyorala K. Validity of clinical diagnosis of heart failure in primary health care. *Eur Heart J* 1991; **12**: 315–321.

22. Carlson KJ, Lee DC-S, Goroll AH et al. An analysis of physicians' reasons for prescribing long-term digitalis therapy in outpatients. *J Chron Dis* 1985; **38**: 733–739.

23. Mattleman SJ, Hakki A-H, Iskandrian AS et al. Reliability of bedside evaluation in determining left ventricular function: correlation with left ventricular ejection fraction determined by radionuclide ventriculagraphy. *J Am Coll Cardiol* 1983; **1**: 417–420.

24. Cease KB, Nicklas JM. Prediction of left ventricular ejection fraction using simple quantitative clinical information. *Am J Med* 1986; **81**: 429–436.

25. Eagle KA, Quertermous T, Singer DE et al. Left ventricular ejection fraction: physician estimates compared with gated blood pool scan measurements. *Arch Intern Med* 1988; **148**: 882–885.

26. McKee PA, Castelli WP, McNamara PM, Kannel WB. The natural history of congestive heart failure: the Framingham study. *N Engl J Med* 1971; **285**: 1441–1446.

The investigation of heart failure

John Byrne

4

The symptoms and physical signs of cardiac failure are non-specific, and clinical assessment is notoriously unreliable (see Chapter 3). Most patients in whom the condition is suspected require further investigation. Heart failure is a clinical syndrome rather than a diagnosis per se and arises through a number of distinct pathophysiological processes. Attention has tended to focus on patients with left ventricular systolic dysfunction, because there are evidence-based treatments for this type of heart failure (ACE inhibitors, beta-blockers, spironolactone). However, heart failure may also develop because of abnormal ventricular filling (so-called diastolic dysfunction), valvular disease, arrhythmias, pericardial disease or metabolic disturbance. This diversity means that there is no easy, all-embracing definition of heart failure, and that no one investigation provides all the answers for each patient. In any case, the scope of investigation extends beyond simply confirming the presence of heart failure. For example, evaluation of pathophysiology, aetiology and prognosis may be relevant in determining the most appropriate management. For example, patients with heart failure who have multivessel coronary artery disease may benefit from revascularization, and surgery is often preferable for patients with valvular disease. Conversely, it may be possible to identify patients with severe heart failure awaiting cardiac transplantation who may respond well to intensified medical therapy.

A further aspect relevant to investigation has emerged recently with the recognition that it is possible to retard or even prevent the development of heart failure. Although chronic heart failure can arise acutely following a major left ventricular insult, the usual onset is more insidious, and often preceded by a latent phase of asymptomatic or minimally symptomatic left ventricular dysfunction. Studies show that the natural history of left ventricular dysfunction is one of relentless deterioration, even without additional ventricular damage.[1] However, the rate of progression can be reduced with early recognition and appropriate drug treatment using ACE inhibitors[1] and perhaps also β-blockers.[2] The implication is that we need to consider strategies for population screening in order to identify 'at risk' individuals who by definition are unlikely to come to medical attention spontaneously. The potential importance of this problem is illustrated by recent work showing that the prevalence of asymptomatic left ventricular dysfunction is likely to be at least as high as that of overt heart failure itself.[3]

The purpose of this chapter is to review the most important investigations available to physicians who manage heart failure, and also to attempt to offer an insight into some of the latest techniques currently being developed.

Core investigations in heart failure

The electrocardiogram

It is mandatory to record a 12-lead electrocardiogram (ECG) in any patient with suspected heart failure if only to exclude tachy- or bradyarrhythmia. However, the ECG may provide other important clues to the presence of significant cardiac disease (see *Figure 4.1*). Pathological Q-waves usually indicate previous myocardial infarction, while increased QRS voltage and ST segment changes are characteristic of left ventricular hypertrophy associated with hypertensive heart disease or aortic stenosis. The presence of bundle branch block does not invariably indicate the presence of significant cardiac disease, but left bundle branch block can be a marker of ventricular dysfunction, while right bundle branch block may be seen in patients with an atrial septal defect. Conversely, a normal 12-lead ECG is unusual in the presence of significant left ventricular dysfunction, and suggests an alternative diagnosis.[4] In other words, whilst an abnormal ECG is relatively non-specific, a normal ECG has useful negative predictive value, and might have a role screening patients with suspected heart failure in primary care. In those with an entirely normal ECG, initial investigations should probably be directed towards finding other causes for their symptoms, such as pulmonary disease.

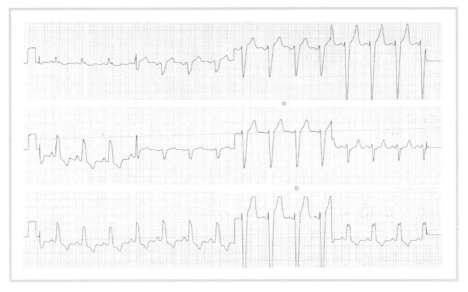

Figure 4.1
The 12-lead electrocardiogram of a 48-year-old man with a dilated cardiomyopathy (left ventricular ejection fraction 18%). There is left bundle branch block, and some evidence of left atrial enlargement.

The chest X-ray

The chest X-ray has traditionally been one of the core investigations of heart failure, and remains important in patients with acute dyspnoea. Its relative importance in chronic heart failure has diminished with the advent of cardiac ultrasound techniques, but its ready availability ensures that it will continue to be requested in many patients (*Figure 4.2*). A number of abnormalities in the cardiac silhouette or in the pulmonary vasculature may provide pointers to cardiac pathology.

Cardiomegaly may indicate dilatation of the cardiac chambers or pericardial effusion. If this is associated with pulmonary oedema or congestion of the upper lobe vessels, then heart failure is likely, although the chest X-ray does not provide a reliable estimate of pulmonary capillary pressure,[5] and correlates poorly with other measures of left ventricular function such as echocardiography.[6] It is extremely important to realise that a normal cardiothoracic ratio does not exclude significant left ventricular systolic dysfunction.

Valvular calcification may be seen in

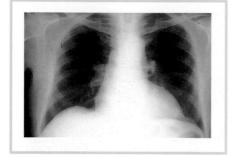

Figure 4.2
Chest X-ray of a patient with chronic heart failure. The patient has been well treated with diuretics and angiotensin converting enzyme inhibitor. The prominent feature is cardiomegaly, with no evidence of pulmonary oedema.

patients with mitral or aortic valve disease, while linear calcification along the pericardial border raises the suspicion of pericardial constriction. Enlargement of the pulmonary arteries may result from shunting of blood through a significant atrial septal defect, and the aortic knuckle may be correspondingly small. Ultimately, however, the most important role of the chest X-ray remains the exclusion of alternative pathology such as pleural effusion, pneumonia, emphysema, tumour or pulmonary fibrosis, all of which may masquerade as heart failure.

Routine blood tests

A number of biochemical and haematological tests may be relevant in the investigation of patients with suspected heart failure.

Measurement of serum electrolytes and hepatic function is important before and after initiation of drug treatment for heart failure. Renal impairment at baseline may be due to renovascular disease, which can be a contraindication to ACE inhibitor therapy. Excessive doses of diuretics may precipitate a deterioration in renal function, and there is also a danger of inducing hypokalaemia or hyponatraemia. Hyponatraemia itself is an ominous feature in patients with established heart failure.[7]

It is important to exclude anaemia as the cause of symptoms in any patient who presents with breathlessness or fatigue, and similarly both hyper- and hypothyroidism can mimic heart failure. Serum ferritin is assayed as a screening test for haemochromatosis in patients with unexplained heart failure, especially if they have diabetes or skin pigmentation, and urinary catecholamine levels provide a method for detecting phaeochromocytoma as a rare cause of dilated cardiomyopathy. Thyroid function should be measured routinely and specific blood tests, such as serum protein electrophoresis, are occasionally indicated.

The echocardiogram

The echocardiogram is the single most important investigation in patients with heart failure (see *Figure 4.3*). A meaningful assessment can be obtained in just a few

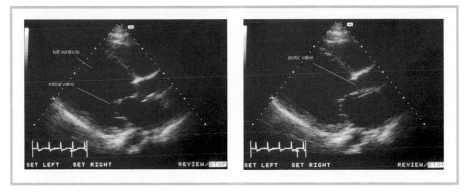

Figure 4.3
The echocardiogram (parasternal long-axis view) of a patient with dilated cardiomyopathy. The left ventricle is dilated and there is very little difference between diastole (mitral valve open, a) and systole (aortic valve open, b).

minutes by an experienced operator allowing real-time estimation of global and regional left ventricular function, while also identifying gross abnormalities of cardiac anatomy including valvular disease. Ultrasound machines are sufficiently portable to allow bedside assessment in casualty departments, in intensive care settings, in the operating theatre, as well as in the cardiology department. Serial examinations can be performed safely in an individual to document the progression of cardiac disease. The main disadvantage is that image quality is poor in a minority of subjects, especially those who are obese or have significant pulmonary disease. Unfortunately, these may be the very patients who are most at risk of having cardiovascular disease.[8]

Echocardiography and ventricular function

Left ventricular function assessment is now the commonest reason for requesting an echocardiogram,[9] and is also the main reason behind the establishment of 'open access' echocardiography services, which allow general practitioners to refer patients with suspected heart failure directly for investigation.[10] The burgeoning popularity of these services is a testament to the widely perceived advantages of the technique. An 'eyeball' assessment of left ventricular contractility takes only a few minutes, and with experience it is possible to provide an accurate estimate of global function which correlates reasonably well with other techniques.[11]

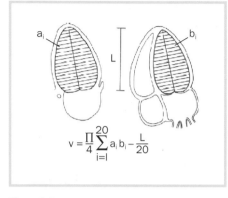

Figure 4.4
Estimating cardiac volume using Simpson's rule. The volume of 20 discs is summed. The left ventricular ejection fraction (LVEF) is derived from the end-diastolic volume (EDV) and end-systolic

$$volume\ (ESV:-\ LVEF = \frac{(EDV-ESV)}{EDV} \times 100\ (\%)$$

A more quantitative assessment is always preferred. Fractional shortening is widely reported as a simple index of ventricular contractility (calculated as the ratio of end-systolic and end-diastolic left ventricular diameters measured at the base of the heart). It is reproducible but can be misleading in patients with regional dysynergy, in whom alternative techniques are to be preferred. The left ventricular ejection fraction (LVEF) is the most widely used index of cardiac function and is recognized as an important prognostic indicator in heart failure.[7,12] It can be derived using a number of different echocardiographic techniques, but the modified Simpson's (disc summation) method is probably the most accurate, especially in patients with regional

wall motion abnormalities[13] (*Figure 4.4*). The technique is time-consuming and technically demanding, but many machines now have on-line analysis packages which facilitate measurements. Reproducibility remains an important problem, however, unless excellent image quality can be obtained, and the suitability of this technique for everyday clinical use is questionable. It should be stressed that there is no universal cut-off ejection fraction value which defines left ventricular dysfunction,[14] although values of 35%[15] and 40%[16] have been used as the entry criteria in some clinical trials.

Another clinically useful method for assessing left ventricular contractility is wall motion analysis, which may provide even greater prognostic information than ejection fraction in heart failure.[17] The ventricle is divided into a number of segments and contractility is assessed individually. The scores are averaged and an overall 'wall motion index' obtained. Recently, a nine-segment model has been used successfully to stratify patients surviving myocardial infarction.[18] A wall motion index of 1.2 or less using this model corresponds approximately to an LVEF of ≤ 35%.

Doppler

Doppler echocardiographic techniques have an important role in evaluating patients with heart failure. Colour flow Doppler readily identifies abnormal valve function or the presence of intracardiac shunts. Quantitative Doppler techniques allow non-invasive measurement of gradients across stenotic valves and estimation of cardiac output, and can be used to obtain an indirect assessment of pulmonary artery pressure. A semiquantitative assessment of valvular regurgitation is also possible, and techniques are still being refined.

Doppler echocardiography can also be used to assess left ventricular diastolic filling using the pattern of early ('E wave') and late ('A wave') inflow through the mitral valve. Abnormal diastolic function is said to be the cause of symptoms in as many as a third of heart failure patients.[19] The E/A ratio is probably the most frequently quoted index of diastolic function, but its value is uncertain.[20] Reversal of the E/A ratio is often assumed to be synonymous with diastolic dysfunction, but in fact is common with increasing age. Conversely, an apparently normal E/A ratio ('pseudo-normalization') may be seen in patients with marked abnormalities of left ventricular filling. A 'restrictive' filling pattern characterized by a short E-wave deceleration time (less than 100 ms) may be more specific, and develops in patients with severe diastolic dysfunction. It indicates a poor prognosis in heart failure patients.[21] Other measures such as intraventricular relaxation time and pulmonary vein flow patterns may also be useful, but most would agree that both the assessment and the management of diastolic dysfunction are less well characterized than those of systolic dysfunction.[22] Some reports question the importance of the diagnosis.[23]

Low-dose dobutamine echocardiography

Dobutamine stress echocardiography (DSE) is now well established as an alternative to nuclear techniques for assessing myocardial ischaemia, but infusion of lower doses of dobutamine (typically 5 to 10 µg/kg per minute) allows assessment of myocardial viability in patients with advanced left ventricular dysfunction.[24]

In many cases ventricular impairment is the result of irreversible myocardial necrosis and scarring. In others there may be areas of viable, but non-contractile myocardium, known as 'hibernating myocardium'. This is thought to occur as a response to chronic ischaemia, or to recurrent episodes of ischaemia. The importance of recognizing the presence of hibernating myocardium is that it can recover contractile function if it is revascularized.[25-27] The best technique for identifying hibernating myocardium is probably positron emission tomography, but its availability is too limited for it to be clinically useful.[28,29]

Low-dose dobutamine echocardiography (LDDE) provides an alternative approach.

Areas of hibernating tissue appear akinetic initially, but begin to contract or thicken as dobutamine is infused, though at higher doses function may again be lost as the tissue becomes more ischaemic. This biphasic response is highly predictive of recovery after revascularization.[30] Hibernating myocardium should be differentiated from 'stunned myocardium', which has superficial similarities. Stunning occurs following a single, transient episode of ischaemia, and myocardial function recovers spontaneously.

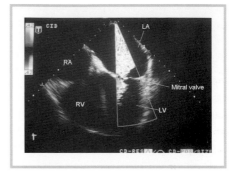

Figure 4.5
Transoesophageal echocardiogram of a patient whose heart failure was due to mitral regurgitation. The left atrium is closest to the transducer (top). The mitral regurgitation is seen as a colour jet from left ventricle to left atrium.

Recent developments in echocardiography

Other techniques promise to extend the role of echocardiography in heart failure still further. Contrast echocardiography employs intravenous contrast agents which cross the pulmonary vascular bed and enter the systemic circulation. Most of these agents contain microbubbles or spheres which reflect ultrasound energy, opacifying the blood pool and so improving endocardial boundary definition. In addition, ultrasound causes these microspheres to resonate at specific harmonic frequencies which can be selectively amplified ('second harmonic imaging') to improve the signal/noise ratio. Contrast echocardiography should make it possible to obtain a quantitative assessment of cardiac function in many patients in whom images were previously considered inadequate. New image processing techniques may soon permit evaluation of myocardial perfusion using these agents, thus providing a direct assessment of coronary patency, and perhaps tissue viability.

Transoesophageal echocardiography

Transoesophageal echocardiography is occasionally valuable in the assessment of patients with heart failure if transthoracic echocardiographic images are inadequate (*Figure 4.5*). It also allows detailed evaluation of structures that may not be seen particularly well using transthoracic imaging, including prosthetic heart valves, the intra-atrial septum and the pulmonary veins.

Ancillary investigations in heart failure

Cardiac catheterization

Cardiac catheterization is rarely if ever required to make the diagnosis of chronic heart failure. However, it has an important part to play in elucidating the aetiology and pathophysiology of heart failure, and it may be valuable in guiding management under certain circumstances.

More than half the patients with left ventricular systolic dysfunction will have underlying coronary artery disease. In some of these patients its presence is suspected because anginal symptoms coexist with heart failure, or because there is a documented history of myocardial infarction. In others, it is detected by stress testing using conventional treadmill or bicycle exercise testing, radionuclide perfusion imaging, or stress echocardiography. In selected patients found to have triple vessel disease, or left main stem stenosis, the prognosis may be improved by successful bypass surgery (*Figure 4.6*). Historically there has been a reluctance to consider conventional revascularization in patients with heart failure and severe ventricular impairment because of the perceived high operative mortality, but this should no longer be the case.

Cardiac catheterization may also provide a useful guide to medical therapy, particularly since physical signs are such an unreliable guide to haemodynamic status.[31] Pulmonary

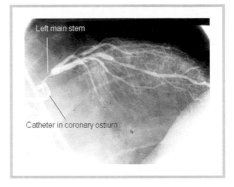

Figure 4.6
Left coronary artery demonstrated during angiography. There is a tight left main stem stenosis.

artery catheterization using a Swan–Ganz catheter is already widely used to optimize filling pressures in patients with acute heart failure and cardiogenic shock. However, it can also be valuable in chronic heart failure, although a certain amount of caution is required in the interpretation of the results. It is important to remember that a normal right heart study does not exclude the diagnosis of heart failure. Pharmacological treatment may normalize filling pressures even in patients with severe heart failure, and indeed this is the aim of 'tailored vasodilator therapy' in which the dosages of diuretics and vasodilators are titrated to achieve predefined haemodynamic targets.[32] This aggressive approach has been shown to improve symptomatic status in patients with end-stage heart failure, even to

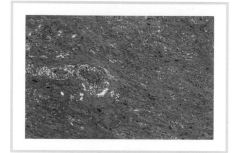

Figure 4.7
Myocardial biopsy specimen from a patient with amyloidosis. Congo red staining has been used and the amyloid deposits show charactersitic red and apple green birefringence under polarized light.

the extent of allowing patients to be taken off the waiting-list for cardiac transplantation.

Other procedures that can be performed at the time of cardiac catheterization include myocardial biopsy in cases where primary myocardial disease (e.g. myocarditis) or infiltrative disease (e.g. amyloid) (*Figure 4.7*) is suspected. Renal angiography may also be considered, particularly in patients with coexistent hypertension, uraemia, or peripheral vascular disease, in whom the prevalence of atheromatous renovascular disease is high.[33] Renal artery stenosis may be a contraindication to ACE inhibitor therapy if it is bilateral, or if the patient has a single functioning kidney. Renal artery stenosis itself may precipitate heart failure, both acute ('flash pulmonary oedema') and chronic.[34] It may be amenable to percutaneous intervention, although the long-term clinical results have

been variable, and the technique is not without hazards.[35]

Nuclear techniques

Blood pool imaging

Nuclear techniques can be useful in assessing ventricular function, especially when echocardiographic images are inadequate or results seem inconsistent. The left ventricular ejection fraction can be obtained using radionuclide ventriculography (also known as multigated acquisition or MUGA scans) in most patients, and regional wall motion can also be evaluated. It offers good reproducibility, and is largely free of the imaging problems faced with echocardiography.

However, there are drawbacks. Gating can be difficult in patients with arrhythmias, particularly atrial fibrillation, and a significant dose of ionizing radiation is administered, limiting the number of studies that can be performed in an individual. Facilities for nuclear cardiology are not as widely available as for echocardiography, and the technique is less convenient to perform. There is a wide variation in the normal range quoted in different institutions, making comparison of results between centres difficult.[36]

Myocardial perfusion imaging

Coronary artery disease is present in the

majority of patients who develop heart failure, and bypass surgery improves the prognosis of those with multivessel coronary disease and ventricular dysfunction. Myocardial perfusion imaging (most commonly using thallium) allows myocardial ischaemia to be recognized in patients with heart failure, and may suggest the need for angiography and revascularization. The technique is more sensitive and specific than treadmill exercise testing, and probably of equivalent predictive accuracy to stress echocardiographic techniques. Myocardial perfusion imaging can also be used to assess myocardial viability in patients with severe ventricular dysfunction being considered for conventional revascularization.[37] It appears to have comparable accuracy to low-dose dobutamine echocardiography for predicting functional recovery following bypass surgery.[38]

Increased lung intake of thallium is sometimes seen in patients with poor left ventricular systolic function and is associated with a poor prognosis.[39]

Exercise testing

Simple treadmill or bicycle exercise provides important information in patients with angina or myocardial infarction, but is not particularly useful for diagnosing heart failure. However, it may demonstrate evidence of underlying cardiac ischaemia, and the addition of cardiopulmonary testing allows measurement of gas exchange (most commonly peak oxygen consumption or VO_2 max), which is widely used as a measure of disease severity and prognosis,[7,12] and increasingly as a guide to the timing of cardiac transplantation.[40] A peak VO_2 of <14 ml/kg/min is considered an indication for heart transplantation in some centres. A fall in arterial oxygen saturation during exercise is unusual in heart failure, and points to pulmonary disease as a possible cause of symptoms.[41]

Ambulatory electrocardiogram

A Holter recording, usually carried out over 24 or 48 hours, does not in itself aid the diagnosis of heart failure, but may identify significant tachy- or brady-arrhythmias, which may be amenable to treatment. Patients with paroxysmal atrial fibrillation, for example, might be considered for anticoagulant therapy. At present, Holter taping is performed for patients with symptoms of palpitations. The recent guidelines from the National Institute of Clinical Excellence suggest that implantable defibrillators should be implanted into all patients with a previous myocardial infarction who have non-sustained ventricular tachycardia on Holter, inducible VT on electrophysiological testing and impaired left ventricular function.[42] Holter recordings will increasingly be seen as part of the routine care of heart failure patients.

Magnetic resonance imaging

Magnetic resonance imaging (MRI) shows great promise for the future. Previously, restricted availability, prolonged imaging protocols and poor patient tolerability had limited its applicability. Recently, however, improvements in technology have dramatically reduced imaging times while improving image quality. The current generation of scanners are capable of real-time cardiac imaging, producing accurate, reproducible measurements of cardiac volumes, cardiac function and muscle mass. Magnetic resonance coronary angiography is not far away as a practical clinical tool, while magnetic resonance renal angiography is already becoming the method of choice for assessing renal vasculature. It is not unrealistic to foresee a time when it will be possible to assess the body's entire vascular tree quickly in a single, non-invasive study. Perhaps even more excitingly MRI will be able to combine this with an assessment of myocardial perfusion and viability.[43]

Computed tomography

Computed tomography (CT) has a relatively minor role in the investigation of patients with heart failure, but again allows accurate assessment of chamber dimensions. It is also a useful technique for demonstrating disease of the pericardium, and in particular pericardial constriction.

Novel investigations in heart failure

Neurohumoral markers

For many years there has been interest in the role of neurohumoral factors in the pathogenesis of heart failure,[44] and this interest intensified with the realization that there might be a role for some of these neurohormones in the diagnosis, assessment and monitoring of heart failure and related conditions.[45] The natriuretic peptides appear to have the greatest potential for clinical use. There are three members of the family of natriuretic peptides altogether, but A-type natriuretic peptide (ANP), and B-type natriuretic peptide (BNP) have been most extensively studied. ANP is secreted primarily from the atria, whereas BNP is predominantly ventricularly derived. Both are synthesized as prohormones, and cleaved into an active C-terminal moiety and a relatively inactive N-terminal fragment (N-ANP and N-BNP, respectively). The N-terminal fragments are cleared more slowly from the circulation than the active C-peptides, and might therefore be expected to provide a better reflection of cardiac status.

At present, however, C-BNP has been the most studied candidate for routine diagnostic use. It is stable in whole blood for several days even at room temperature, which facilitates handling and processing.[46] It is superior to other neurohormones for diagnosing left ventricular dysfunction and predicting prognosis in heart failure,[47] and after myocardial infarction.[48] It has been used to establish whether there is a cardiac cause of breathlessness in patients in the community,[49] and in patients presenting acutely to hospital.[50] It may also have an important role in screening of the wider population in order to identify patients with asymptomatic left ventricular dysfunction[51,52] who may benefit from the early use of ACE inhibitors. Where availability of cardiac imaging is limited, C-BNP might be used as an initial screening test to determine which patients should have an echocardiogram. Finally, there is preliminary evidence that it might have a part to play in guiding drug therapy, and monitoring the response to treatment.[53,54]

Autonomic function assessment

Heart failure is associated with abnormalities of autonomic activity which may be of value in predicting prognosis. As well as an increase in sympathetic nervous system activity there is decreased parasympathetic tone. This may be evident even in the early stages of heart failure, and is reflected in reduced heart rate variability and impaired baroreflex sensitivity (measures of tonic and reflex parasympathetic activity, respectively). The clinical importance of techniques that measure these variables is as yet uncertain.

Conclusion

Although a growing number of tools are at the disposal of the physician investigating and managing patients with suspected heart failure, the key is still thorough clinical evaluation combined with simple baseline investigations. The negative predictive value of a normal 12-lead ECG should be more widely appreciated, since it may allow more selective referral for cardiac investigation. Beyond this, echocardiography is the cornerstone of investigation, as it provides a comprehensive, non-invasive assessment of global cardiac function. For the majority of patients this is sufficient to confirm the diagnosis, but if doubt remains there are a range of other techniques available.

The challenge that faces us now is to refine our approach so that patients can be recognized earlier in the course of their disease. If appropriate effective treatment can be offered more quickly, we may delay or even prevent the development of overt heart failure. This is no idle dream. In the near future, humoral markers may be used to screen for the presence of left ventricular dysfunction in the community, while MRI will offer a more precise evaluation of all aspects of cardiac pathophysiology, perhaps replacing echocardiography, nuclear techniques and even angiography. The future of heart failure investigation looks exciting indeed.

References

1. Konstam MA, Kronenberg MW, Rousseau MF et al. Effects of the angiotensin converting enzyme inhibitor enalapril on the long-term progression of left ventricular dilatation in patients with asymptomatic systolic dysfunction. SOLVD (Studies of Left Ventricular Dysfunction) Investigators. *Circulation* 1993; **88**: 2277–2283.

2. Colucci WS, Packer M, Bristow MR et al. Carvedilol inhibits clinical progression in patients with mild symptoms of heart failure. US Carvedilol Heart Failure Study Group. *Circulation* 1996; **94**: 2800–2806.

3. McDonagh TA, Morrison CE, Lawrence A et al. Symptomatic and asymptomatic left-ventricular systolic dysfunction in an urban population. *Lancet* 1997; **350**: 829–833.

4. Davie AP, Francis CM, Love MP et al. Value of the electrocardiogram in identifying heart failure due to left ventricular systolic dysfunction. *Br Med J* 1996; **312**: 222.

5. Chakko S, Woska D, Martinez H et al. Clinical, radiographic, and hemodynamic correlations in chronic congestive heart failure: conflicting results may lead to inappropriate care. *Am J Med* 1991; **90**: 353–359.

6. Clark AL, Coats AJ. Unreliability of cardiothoracic ratio as a marker of left ventricular impairment: comparison with radionuclide ventriculography and echocardiography. *Postgrad Med J* 2000; **76**: 289–291.

7. Parameshwar J, Keegan J, Sparrow J et al. Predictors of prognosis in severe chronic heart failure. *Am Heart J* 1992; **123**: 421–426.

8. Kober L, Torp-Pedersen C. Clinical characteristics and mortality of patients screened for entry into the Trandolapril Cardiac Evaluation (TRACE) study. *Am J Cardiol* 1995; **76**: 1–5.

9. Gillespie ND, Struthers AD, Pringle SD. Changing echocardiography request patterns between 1988 and 1993. *Health Bull* 1996; **54**: 395–401.

10. Francis CM, Caruana L, Kearney P et al. Open access echocardiography in management of heart failure in the community. *Br Med J* 1995; **310**: 634–636.

11. Willenheimer RB, Israelsson BA, Cline CMJ, Erhardt LR. Simplified echocardiography in the diagnosis of heart failure. *Scand Cardiovasc J* 1997; **31**: 8–16.

12. Cohn JN, Johnson GR, Shabetai R et al. Ejection fraction, peak exercise oxygen consumption, cardiothoracic ratio, ventricular arrhythmias, and plasma norepinephrine as determinants of prognosis in heart failure. The V-HeFT VA Cooperative Studies Group. *Circulation* 1993; **87**: V15–V16.

13. Schiller NB, Shah PM, Crawford M et al. Recommendations for quantitation of the left ventricle by two-dimensional echocardiography. American Society of Echocardiography Committee on Standards, Subcommittee on Quantitation of Two-Dimensional Echocardiograms. *J Am Soc Echocardiogr* 1989; **2**: 358–367.

14. Ray SG, Metcalfe MJ, Oldroyd KG et al. Do radionuclide and echocardiographic techniques give a universal cut off value for left ventricular ejection fraction that can be used to select patients for treatment with ACE inhibitors after myocardial infarction? *Br Heart J* 1995; **73**: 466–469.

15. The SOLVD Investigators. Effect of enalapril on survival in patients with reduced left ventricular ejection fractions and congestive

heart failure. *N Engl J Med* 1991; **325:** 293–302.

16. Pfeffer MA, Braunwald E, Moye LA et al. Effect of captopril on mortality and morbidity in patients with left ventricular dysfunction after myocardial infarction. Results of the survival and ventricular enlargement trial. *N Engl J Med* 1992; **327:** 669–677.

17. Madsen BK, Videbaek R, Stokholm H et al. Prognostic value of echocardiography in 190 patients with chronic congestive heart failure. A comparison with New York Heart Association functional classes and radionuclide ventriculography. *Cardiology* 1996; **87:** 250–256.

18. Kober L, Torp-Pedersen C, Carlsen J et al. An echocardiographic method for selecting high risk patients shortly after acute myocardial infarction, for inclusion in multi-centre studies (as used in the TRACE study). *Eur Heart J* 1994; **15:** 1616–1620.

19. Cohn JN, Johnson G. Heart failure with normal ejection fraction. The V-HeFT Study. Veterans Administration Cooperative Study Group. *Circulation* 1990; **81:** III48–III53.

20. Davie AP, Francis CM, Caruana L et al. The prevalence of left ventricular diastolic filling abnormalities in patients with suspected heart failure. *Eur Heart J* 1997; **18:** 981–984.

21. Giannuzzi P, Temporelli PL, Bosimini E et al. Independent and incremental prognostic value of Doppler-derived mitral deceleration time of early filling in both symptomatic and asymptomatic patients with left ventricular dysfunction. *J Am Coll Cardiol* 1996; **28:** 383–390.

22. Vasan RS, Benjamin EJ, Levy D. Congestive heart failure with normal left ventricular systolic function. Clinical approaches to the diagnosis and treatment of diastolic heart failure. *Arch Intern Med* 1996; **156:** 146–157.

23. Caruana L, Petrie MC, Davie AP, McMurray JJV. Do patients with suspected heart failure and preserved left ventricular systolic function suffer from 'diastolic heart failure' or from misdiagnosis? A prospective descriptive study. *Br Med J* 2000; **321:** 215–218.

24. La Canna G, Alfieri O, Giubbini R et al. Echocardiography during infusion of dobutamine for identification of reversible dysfunction in patients with chronic coronary artery disease. *J Am Coll Cardiol* 1994; **23:** 617–626.

25. Rahimtoola SH. The hibernating myocardium. *Am Heart J* 1989; **117:** 211–221.

26. Wijns W, Vatner SF, Camici PG. Hibernating myocardium. *N Engl J Med* 1998; **339:** 173–181.

27. Bax JJ, Poldermans D, Elhendy A et al. Improvement of left ventricular ejection fraction, heart failure symptoms and prognosis after revascularization in patients with chronic coronary artery disease and viable myocardium detected by dobutamine stress echocardiography. *J Am Coll Cardiol* 1999; **34:** 163–169.

28. Di Carli MF, Asgarzadie F, Schelbert HR et al. Quantitative relation between myocardial viability and improvement in heart failure symptoms after revascularization in patients with ischemic cardiomyopathy. *Circulation* 1995; **92:** 3436–3444.

29. Pagano D, Bonser RS, Townend JN et al. Predictive value of dobutamine echocardiography and positron emission tomography in identifying hibernating myocardium in patients with postischaemic heart failure. *Heart* 1998; **79:** 281–288.

30. Cornel JH, Bax JJ, Elhendy A et al. Biphasic response to dobutamine predicts

improvement of global left ventricular function after surgical revascularization in patients with stable coronary artery disease: implications of time course of recovery on diagnostic accuracy. *J Am Coll Cardiol* 1998; **31**: 1002–1010.

31. Stevenson LW, Perloff JK. The limited reliability of physical signs for estimating hemodynamics in chronic heart failure. *J Am Med Assoc* 1989; **26**: 884–888.

32. Steimle AE, Stevenson LW, Chelimsky-Fallick C et al. Sustained hemodynamic efficacy of therapy tailored to reduce filling pressures in survivors with advanced heart failure. *Circulation* 1997; **96**: 1165–1172.

33. Greco BA, Breyer JA. The natural history of renal artery stenosis: who should be evaluated for suspected ischemic nephropathy? *Semin Nephrol* 1996; **16**: 2–11.

34. Missouris CG, Belli AM, MacGregor GA. 'Apparent' heart failure: a syndrome caused by renal artery stenoses. *Heart* 2000; **83**: 152–155.

35. Weibull H, Bergqvist D, Jonsson K et al. Analysis of complications after percutaneous transluminal angioplasty of renal artery stenoses. *Eur J Vasc Surg* 1987; **1**: 77–84.

36. Underwood R, Gibson C, Tweddel A, Flint J. A survey of nuclear cardiological practice in Great Britain. The British Nuclear Cardiology Group. *Br Heart J* 1992; **67**: 273–277.

37. Ragosta M, Beller GA, Watson DD et al. Quantitative planar rest-redistribution 201Tl imaging in detection of myocardial viability and prediction of improvement in left ventricular function after coronary bypass surgery in patients with severely depressed left ventricular function. *Circulation* 1993; **87**: 1630–1641.

38. Vanoverschelde JL, D'Hondt AM, Marwick T et al. Head-to-head comparison of exercise–redistribution–reinjection thallium single-photon emission computed tomography and low dose dobutamine echocardiography for prediction of reversibility of chronic left ventricular ischemic dysfunction. *J Am Coll Cardiol* 1996; **28**: 432–442.

39. O'Rouke RA. Lung uptake of thallium as a prognostic indicator. *N Engl J Med* 1987; **317**: 1532–1534.

40. Mancini DM, Eisen H, Kussmaul W et al. Value of peak exercise oxygen consumption for optimal timing of cardiac transplantation in ambulatory patients with heart failure. *Circulation* 1991; **83**: 778–786.

41. Clark AL, Coats AJ. Usefulness of arterial blood gas estimations during exercise in patients with chronic heart failure. *Br Heart J* 1994; **71**: 528–530.

42. Guidance on the use of implantable cardioverter debrillators for arrhythmias. National Institute for Clinical Excellence. London, September 2000.

43. Sensky PR, Jivan A, Hudson NM et al. Coronary artery disease: combined stress MR imaging protocol-one-stop evaluation of myocardial perfusion and function. *Radiology* 2000; **215**: 608–614.

44. Packer M. The neurohormonal hypothesis: a theory to explain the mechanism of disease progression in heart failure. *J Am Coll Cardiol* 1992; **20**: 248–254.

45. Francis GS, Cohn JN, Johnson G et al. Plasma norepinephrine, plasma renin activity, and congestive heart failure. Relations to survival and the effects of therapy in V-HeFT II. The V-HeFT VA Cooperative Studies Group. *Circulation* 1993; **87**: VI40–VI48.

46. Murdoch DR, Byrne J, Morton JJ et al. Brain natriuretic peptide is stable in whole blood and can be measured using a simple rapid assay: implications for clinical practice. *Heart* 1997; **78**: 594–597.

47. Tsutamoto T, Wada A, Maeda K et al. Plasma brain natriuretic peptide level as a biochemical marker of morbidity and mortality in patients with asymptomatic or minimally symptomatic left ventricular dysfunction. Comparison with plasma angiotensin II and endothelin-1. *Eur Heart J* 1999; **20**: 1799–1807.

48. Richards AM, Nicholls MG, Yandle TG et al. Neuroendocrine prediction of left ventricular function and heart failure after acute myocardial infarction. *Heart* 1999; **81**: 114–120.

49. Cowie MR, Struthers AD, Wood DA et al. Value of natriuretic peptides in assessment of patients with possible new heart failure in primary care. *Lancet* 1997; **350**: 1349–1353.

50. Davis M, Espiner E, Richards G et al. Plasma brain natriuretic peptide in assessment of acute dyspnoea. *Lancet* 1994; **343**: 440–444.

51. McDonagh TA, Robb SD, Murdoch DR et al. Biochemical detection of left-ventricular systolic dysfunction. *Lancet* 1998; **351**: 9–13.

52. Smith H, Pickering RM, Struthers A et al. Biochemical diagnosis of ventricular dysfunction in elderly patients in general practice: observational study. *Br Med J* 2000; **320**: 906–908.

53. Murdoch DR, McDonagh TA, Byrne J et al. Titration of vasodilator therapy in chronic heart failure according to plasma brain natriuretic peptide concentration: randomized comparison of the hemodynamic neuroendocrine effects of tailored versus empirical therapy. *Am Heart J* 1999; **138**: 1126–1132.

54. Troughton RW, Frampton CM, Yandle TG et al. Treatment of heart failure guided by plasma aminoterminal brain natriuretic peptide (N-BNP) concentrations. *Lancet* 2000; **355**: 1126–1130.

Treatment: diuretics

Mark C Petrie

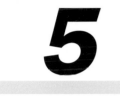

Diuretics have been the mainstay of chronic heart failure therapy for decades. During the 1990s newer agents, such as angiotensin converting enzyme (ACE) inhibitors and, more recently, β-blockers, have diverted attention from this commonly used drug class.

Rationale for diuretic therapy in heart failure

Diuretics are used to counteract one of the hallmarks of the syndrome of chronic heart failure: sodium and water retention. Decreased cardiac output and increased arterial resistance result in decreased renal blood flow and glomerular filtration rate.[1] Neurohumoral activation occurs in response to a reduction in tissue perfusion. These neurohumoral pathways have profound renal effects and are activated to maintain organ perfusion and kidney function. For example, angiotensin II, by acting as a vasoconstrictor at the efferent glomerular arteriole, increases filtration fraction, preserving glomerular filtration rate in the face of a fall in renal plasma flow. The renin-angiotensin-aldosterone (RAAS), sympathetic nervous system (SNS) and arginine vasopressin (antidiuretic hormone, AVP or ADH) also cause sodium and water retention. The resulting sodium and water retaining state is expressed clinically by oedema, pulmonary crackles, hepatomegaly with ascites and raised jugular venous pressure. Diuretics are employed to increase renal sodium excretion with concurrent improvement of these clinical features. This usually occurs, however, at the cost of further neurohumoral activation.

Classes of diuretics

Loop diuretics

This is the most widely used class of diuretics in the management of heart failure. Loop diuretics are actively excreted into the tubular lumen, where they cause a potent diuresis by blocking active chloride transport from the thick ascending limb of the loop of Henle

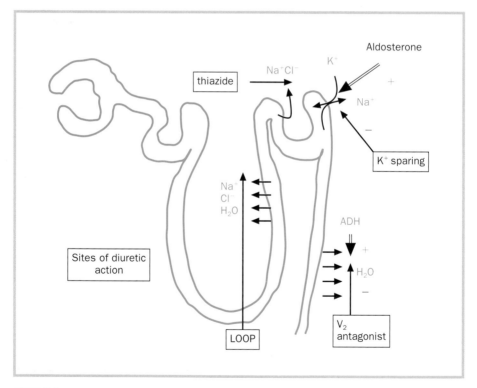

Figure 5.1
Sites of diuretic action in the nephron. Loop diuretics function in the thick ascending loop of Henle, thiazides in the distal convoluted tubule, as do potassium sparing diuretics. V_2 antagonists work in the collecting duct.

(*Figure 5.1*), which normally cotransports sodium and water out of the renal tubule. When a loop diuretic is given, sodium and water are lost with chloride. The potency of loop diuretics is a result of their site of action. The ascending loop of Henle is responsible for reabsorbing 25% of filtered sodium and water from the 180 litres of glomerular filtrate/day

The two commonly used loop diuretics are frusemide and bumetanide. A dose of frusemide of 40 mg is approximately equivalent to a dose of bumetanide of 1 mg. Gastrointestinal absorption of frusemide can be altered and may be unpredictable in patients with heart failure, particularly when oedema and hepatomegaly are present. Bumetanide absorption is less affected than frusemide and, in addition, food has less effect on the absorption of bumetanide than frusemide.[2] Frusemide has approximately 40% bioavailability, whereas bumetanide has around 80%.

The newer loop diuretic torasemide has some theoretical advantages over more traditional diuretics. It has more predictable bioavailability (around 90%) and less renal excretion (20% (80% hepatic) in comparison to 100% for frusemide). It also causes less potassium loss.[3] A particular advantage in the elderly is that the diuresis induced by torasemide is less brisk than with the better known agents.

Thiazide diuretics

Thiazides are less potent than loop diuretics, reflecting their site of action. They act on the cortical diluting segment, which is responsible for reabsorbing 10–15% of the filtered sodium load (*Figure 5.1*). They have a more prolonged action (up to 72 hours) but do not provide broad dose–response ranges. They tend to be used in the later stages of heart failure in combination with loop diuretics (see later). Thiazide diuretics are less effective in patients with renal dysfunction. The most commonly used thiazide is bendrofluazide.

Metolazone

Metolazone is a thiazide diuretic. Although it was historically thought to have important actions on the proximal tubule, the additive response when used in combination with a loop diuretic has been demonstrated to be due to actions at the distal nephron (*Figure 5.1*).[4,5] Recent evidence suggests that metolazone is not superior to other thiazides when used in combination with loop diuretics. Metolazone remains effective in patients with renal impairment of at least moderate severity.

Potassium-sparing diuretics

These drugs act on the distal tubule, where sodium is reabsorbed in exchange for potassium or hydrogen (*Figure 5.1*). By inhibiting this process, sodium is excreted and potassium retained. Different agents have different mechanisms of action.

Spironolactone

Spironolactone is a competitive aldosterone inhibitor. Until recently spironolactone was most commonly used in the management of resistant heart failure in combination with loop and thiazide diuretics. The publication of the RALES trial in 1999 has, however, dramatically altered the role of spironolactone in the management of chronic heart failure.[6] This landmark trial randomized patients with markedly symptomatic chronic stable heart failure (patients had to have been classified as NYHA IV within 6 months of randomization), already receiving ACE inhibitors and loop diuretics, to low-dose spironolactone or placebo. Patients on spironolactone showed improved all cause mortality (27% risk reduction, $p < 0.0001$). A reduction in hospitalizations for cardiac causes (30% risk reduction) and, in particular, for worsening chronic heart failure (35% risk reduction) was also found. The mean daily dose after 24 months' follow-up was only 26 mg (previously doses of 50–200 mg had been used in refractory heart failure as additive therapy).

There was a remarkably low incidence of hyperkalaemia. Serious hyperkalaemia occurred in only 1.7% of the spironolactone group in comparison to 1.2% of the placebo group.

However, patients were included only if their serum creatinine concentration was < 221 μmol/l. Close monitoring of participants' serum potassium concentrations was undertaken (weeks 1, 4, 5, 8, 12, etc.). There is some concern that this low rate of hyperkalaemia may not translate to routine clinical practice, although evidence for this thus far is only anecdotal.

The RALES trial results are often interpreted as demonstrating the benefits of aldosterone antagonism. These data could, however, equally well be taken as demonstrating the benefits of additional diuretic therapy. The design of the study did not include a limb with an additional, non-aldosterone antagonist diuretic, such as amiloride. It is not certain, therefore, that aldosterone antagonism per se was the reason for the improved outcome. However, the dose of spironolactone has been shown in a pilot study to have no measurable effect on sodium and water excretion/body weight.

The diuretic effects of spironolactone continue for markedly longer than that of loop diuretics, lasting for up to 2–3 days. The other adverse effect associated with spironolactone was that of gynaecomastia in approximately 10% of men.[6]

Amiloride

Amiloride directly inhibits sodium transport. In practice, amiloride is usually used when hypokalaemia occurs in association with the more potent loop or thiazide diuretics. The diuretic effect of amiloride persists for about 24 hours.

Adverse effects of diuretics

These are predominantly electrolyte and metabolic disorders. The reported incidence is anywhere from 14 to 60%.[7]

Hypokalaemia

Both loop and thiazide diuretics cause potassium depletion, to which chronic heart failure patients are already predisposed, because of neurohumoral activation. Thiazides are the most frequent offenders.[8,9] Hypokalaemia predisposes to life-threatening arrhythmias and increases the risk of digitalis toxicity (and toxicity from other potentially arrhythmogenic drugs such as tricyclic antidepressants, phenothiazines and antiarrhythmic agents). As high-grade ventricular arrhythmias and sudden death are frequently observed in chronic heart failure, potassium depletion must be avoided.

Hyperkalaemia

Potassium-sparing diuretics can cause hyperkalaemia (see spironolactone). It should be remembered that these agents are often found in combination tablets such as co-amilofruse (e.g. Frumil®).

Hyponatraemia

Hyponatraemia is commonly seen in patients with severe chronic heart failure on long-term diuretic therapy. It is a poor prognostic marker.[10] Thiazides cause hyponatraemia more frequently than loop diuretics.

Hypomagnesaemia

Magnesium depletion is common in patients on long-term diuretic therapy. Tissue magnesium depletion may occur without a reduction in serum magnesium concentration (this occurs only in advanced, severe deficiency). Hypomagnesaemia, like hypokalaemia, predisposes to ventricular arrhythmias. It may be impossible to correct potassium deficiency unless magnesium deficiency is corrected first. Potassium-conserving diuretics also conserve magnesium.

Other metabolic/electrolyte disturbances

Hypocalcaemia, hyperuricaemia and metabolic alkalosis also occur with long-term diuretic therapy. Thiazide diuretics can alter glucose metabolism and can precipitate diabetes mellitus. Gout is a particularly difficult problem in patients with chronic heart failure as non-steroidal anti-inflammatory drugs (NSAIDs) cause sodium and water retention, renal impairment and counteract the effect of diuretics. Colchicine is the preferred treatment.

Other adverse effects

High-dose intravenous frusemide can cause deafness.

Correction of electrolyte depletion

Hypokalaemia

There is no place for oral potassium supplementation in heart failure. Potassium supplements are ineffective at preventing potassium depletion and are unpleasant to take. In addition, they can cause upper and lower gastrointestinal tract erosion and even perforation.

Potassium-sparing diuretics should be given if hypokalaemia occurs. These are effective in maintaining concentrations of serum potassium, serum magnesium and total body potassium.[11] The complicating factor is that every patient with left ventricular systolic dysfunction should be taking an ACE inhibitor unless there is genuine intolerance to these agents. ACE inhibitors, like potassium-sparing diuretics, cause potassium retention and predispose to hyperkalaemia. Many patients do not need potassium-sparing diuretics once they are established on an ACE inhibitor, and it is important to monitor potassium throughout. Patients with severe heart failure, and perhaps all those patients needing potassium-sparing agents, should be given low-dose spironolactone,[6] again with regular monitoring of potassium. If a patient is taking a combination diuretic (e.g. Frumil), it should be changed to the pure loop diuretic (e.g. frusemide) before an ACE inhibitor is given.

For more severe potassium depletion, intravenous administration is recommended. Patients require 40–120 mmol to maintain potassium homeostasis. It is important to remember that hypokalaemia may persist until magnesium deficiency is corrected. Magnesium is a cofactor in the sodium/potassium ATPase pump. Only 1% of magnesium is found extracellularly, so serum and urinary concentrations do not accurately reflect the total body content.

Hyponatraemia

Only water restriction contributes to correcting this electrolyte abnormality at present though AVP antagonists may be useful in the future. Water, diluted drinks (e.g. fruit drinks diluted with water) should be avoided and a 1.0–1.5 l fluid restriction (milk, tea, coffee) imposed.

Hypomagnesaemia

This should be corrected by intravenous infusion, especially when patients on long-term diuretic therapy suffer ventricular arrhythmias.

Who should receive treatment with a diuretic?

Diuretics should be used in patients with evidence of sodium and water retention (pulmonary or peripheral oedema) in the presence of left ventricular systolic dysfunction. Breathless patients with chronic heart failure without these signs also show a better symptomatic response to diuretics than to any other treatment.[12,13]

Do diuretics work?

Diuretics improve the symptoms and signs of fluid overload in chronic heart failure.[14] Indeed, symptomatic improvement is unmatched by any other drug class alone.[12] These effects are seen in everyday clinical experience, although they have been formally documented in only a few small placebo controlled trials with loop diuretics.[15,16] The sparse data available suggest that loop and thiazide diuretics are equally efficacious in mild chronic heart failure, and that loop diuretics are more effective in more severe chronic heart failure.[8,9]

Are angiotensin converting enzyme inhibitors a substitute for diuretics?

Every patient with left ventricular systolic dysfunction, whether symptomatic or not, should receive an ACE inhibitor. The advent of ACE inhibitors led to suggestions that they could replace diuretics. They have, however, been shown to be inadequate substitutes for diuretics, at least in patients with a history of pulmonary oedema. One trial suggested that, if patients have mildly impaired left ventricular dysfunction, are on the equivalent of frusemide 40 mg/day and have no history of systemic hypertension or pulmonary oedema, substituting a diuretic with an ACE inhibitor may be warranted.[17]

In mild heart failure, thiazide diuretics and ACE inhibitors appear to be equally effective.[18] For patients presenting with no signs of fluid retention, but otherwise symptomatic left ventricular systolic dysfunction (e.g. breathlessness on exertion), it is reasonable to withhold diuretics for a month to determine whether an ACE inhibitor alone can relieve their symptoms. For patients with moderately severe heart failure, controlled trials suggest that increasing the dose of diuretic and adding an ACE inhibitor are equally effective in improving symptoms and exercise capacity (though an ACE inhibitor is essential in order to improve prognosis).[19,20]

Are diuretics an 'evidence-based' therapy?

In the modern era of evidence-based cardiology, diuretics are frustrating. While the efficacy of diuretics in relieving symptoms of sodium and water retention is evident in everyday clinical experience, few large-scale trials have addressed hard end-points, such as mortality.[6] Such trials are impractical, as diuretics are indispensable in the management of chronic heart failure and indeed diuretics are on the whole relatively inexpensive and therefore unattractive to pharmaceutical companies. These factors make the RALES trial all the more remarkable.[6]

Do diuretics influence the pathophysiology of chronic heart failure?

All types of diuretic cause neuroendocrine stimulation. Frusemide has been shown to cause both acute and chronic stimulation of the sympathetic and renin–angiotensin–aldosterone systems.[14,21–24] Neuroendocrine activation predicts a worse outcome in chronic heart failure, so diuretics may have a negative effect on long-term outcome. This is currently, however, an academic question, as there are no alternative drugs for alleviating fluid and water retention in chronic heart failure. It has been suggested that these potential adverse neuroendocrine and

haemodynamic changes may to some extent be countered by treatment with an ACE inhibitor. Perhaps a new generation of diuretics, if developed, may allow future comparisons of effects on pathophysiology and other clinically relevant end-points.

Practical management issues

Role of dietary sodium/fluid restriction

The clinical effectiveness of diuretics depends upon adherence to a low sodium diet.[25] Patients should be instructed to limit their daily intake of sodium to 2.5 g/day, although this can be further reduced depending on the severity of the oedema. Patient should be encouraged to limit their fluid intake to around 1.5 l/day.

Self-weighing

Patients should weigh themselves on a regular basis. When there is more than 0.5 kg in weight gain over a period of a week patients should be instructed to increase their diuretics, for example by 40 mg of frusemide, for 4–5 days. Such instructions are best suited where provisions for contact with specialist services (for example specialist heart failure nurses) are available.

Day-to-day use of diuretics

We commonly employ loop diuretics from the start of treatment. Our rationale is that the shallow dose–response curves of thiazide diuretics do not allow dose titration as the syndrome progresses. This precludes their use as single agents. The effective dose of frusemide is usually 40 mg/day or bumetanide 1 mg. A dose of 80–120 mg of frusemide may be necessary. If a greater dose of diuretic is needed, repeated rather than larger doses should be used. Before increasing doses above 120 mg twice a day, the preferred approach is to add another diuretic with a different site of action on the nephron.

Management of diuretic resistance

Diuretic resistance is the condition of increasing symptoms of fluid and electrolyte retention in the face of increased doses of diuretics. Several therapeutic interventions can be used to stimulate appropriate diuresis. Intravenous diuretics are useful in this situation, and are more efficacious than oral diuretics in patients with fluid retention due to impaired absorption of oral diuretic from an oedematous small bowel. The dosage should be escalated until the desired effect is produced. An ultrahigh dose of loop diuretic may be effective,[26] but large doses of frusemide can cause deafness. Continuous intravenous infusion of loop diuretics also increases their effectiveness.[27]

An alternative is the use of combinations of diuretics that act at different sites of the nephron (for example a thiazide and a loop diuretic combined – so called 'sequential nephron blockade').[28] Such strategies can cause an unpredictably large diuresis, leading to intravascular dehydration, hypotension, severe electrolyte upset and renal failure. Close monitoring of electrolytes and renal function is necessary. Further options for refractory oedema (normally with concurrent renal failure) are dialysis, haemofiltration and ultrafiltration.[29–31]

Drug interactions

Non-steroidal anti-inflammatory drugs

Non-steroidal anti-inflammatory drugs (NSAIDs) blunt the natriuretic effect of diuretics by poorly understood mechanisms.[32] NSAIDs may also cause renal dysfunction and hyperkalaemia in patients taking potassium-sparing diuretics and ACE inhibitors. It is increasingly recognized that NSAIDs can worsen or precipitate chronic heart failure, especially in the elderly.[33]

Digoxin

Diuretic-induced hypokalaemia can predispose to digitoxicity.

Advice to patients and carers

All diuretics cause inconvenience for chronic heart failure sufferers. They usually have to organize their daily activities around the period of most intense diuresis. Loop diuretics may often be preferred, as their effect usually diminishes 4 hours after the dose. Thiazides can cause problems with nocturia. Patients should be informed that there is generally no fixed time that the diuretic should be taken. When a diuretic is prescribed twice a day it is important to emphasize that it should not be taken last thing at night. Consideration should be given to patient mobility and toilet logistics.

Possible future diuretics

There has not been a new therapeutic agent available in the management of sodium and water retention for decades. However, improved understanding of the neurohumoral derangement in heart failure has provided potential candidates.

Natriuretic peptides and neutral endopeptidase inhibitors

An encouraging profile of natriuresis, diuresis, suppression of the renin–angiotensin–aldosterone system and vasodilatation suggests that A-type natriuretic peptide (ANP) and B-type natriuretic peptide (BNP) may be appropriate treatments for chronic heart failure. While these agents when infused intravenously do cause a degree of diuresis in heart failure patients, the lack of orally active preparations has limited their investigation. An alternative approach is the use of neutral endopeptidase inhibitors. These agents inhibit the breakdown of natriuretic peptides by neutral endopeptidase. By inhibiting the breakdown of ANP and BNP, the rationale is that increased plasma concentrations should mediate beneficial results. Although some success in improving morbidity in chronic heart failure has been found, neutral endopeptidase inhibitors are not clinically effective diuretics.[34] As well as metabolizing natriuretic peptides, neutral endopeptidase also metabolizes endothelin and angiotensin II. Neutral endopeptidase inhibitors could also therefore potentiate the vasoconstrictor, antinatriuretic effects of these peptides and this might explain the lack of diuresis produced. An encouraging recent development is that of an orally available combined neutral endopeptidase/ACE inhibitor, omapatrilat. The primary effects of this agent appear to be hypotensive rather than diuretic. Its use in chronic heart failure is currently being evaluated in the OVERTURE study.

Arginine vasopressin antagonists

The final target in the nephron for increasing urine loss is the collecting duct. Vasopressin (or antidiuretic hormone) mediates fluid retention via V_2 receptors in the collecting duct, causing water channels to open and water to pass from the collecting duct into the renal medulla by osmosis. Vasopressin antagonists in development block the V_2 receptor, thus promoting an aquaresis (there is no net sodium loss through this mechanism). In studies of normal subjects, V_2 antagonists cause a profound aquaresis. They offer potentially important benefits for heart failure patients, particularly those who have hyponatraemia, and those who have developed diuretic resistance.

Conclusions

Diuretics remain central to modern heart failure management. Careful use of appropriate doses, together with monitoring to avoid adverse events, allows the relief of symptoms of sodium and water retention in chronic heart failure. Although their effect on the syndrome of heart failure is uncertain, they will remain necessary in their current form until a new generation of agents capable of relieving sodium and water retention is developed.

References

1. Cody RJ, Ljungman S, Covit AB et al. Regulation of glomerular-filtration rate in chronic congestive heart-failure patients. *Kidney Int* 1988; **34**: 361–367.

2. McCrindle JL, Wa TC, Barron W, Prescott LF. Effect of frusemide on the absorption of frusemide and bumetanide in man. *Br J Clin Pharmacol* 1996; **42**: 743–746.

3. Dunn CJ, Fitton A, Brogden RN. Torasemide—an update of its pharmacological properties and therapeutic efficacy. *Drugs* 1995; **49**: 121–142.

4. Oster JR, Epstein M, Smoller S. Combined therapy with thiazide-type and loop diuretic agents for resistant sodium retention. *Ann Intern Med* 1983; **99**: 405–406.

5. Brater DC, Pressley RH, Anderson SA. Mechanisms of the synergistic combination of metolazone and bumetanide. *J Pharmacol Exp Ther* 1985; **233**: 70–74.

6. Pitt B, Zannad F, Remme WJ et al. The effect of spironolactone on morbidity and mortality in patients with severe heart failure. *N Engl J Med* 1999; **341**: 709–717.

7. Cody RJ, Pickworth KK. Approaches to diuretic therapy and electrolyte imblance in congestive heart failure. In: Deedwania PC (ed). *Update in Congestive Heart Failure*. Philadelphia: WB Saunders, 1994.

8. Pehrsson SK. Multicenter comparison between slow-release furosemide and bendroflumethiazide in congestive heart-failure. *Eur J Clin Pharmacol* 1985; **28**: 235–239.

9. Vermeulen A, Chadha DR. Slow-release furosemide and hydrochlorothiazide in congestive cardiac-failure—a controlled trial. *J Clin Pharmacol* 1982; **22**: 513–519.

10. Lee WH, Packer M. Prognostic importance of serum sodium concentration and its modification by converting-enzyme inhibition in patients with severe chronic heart-failure. *Circulation* 1986; **73**: 257–267.

11. Kohvakka A. Maintenance of potassium-balance during long-term diuretic therapy in chronic heart-failure patients with thiazide-induced hypokalemia—comparison of potassium supplementation with potassium-chloride and potassium-sparing agents, amiloride and triamterene. *Int J Clin Pharmacol Ther* 1988; **26**: 273–277.

12. Richardson A, Scriven AJ, PooleWilson PA et al. Double-blind comparison of captopril alone against frusemide plus amiloride in mild heart-failure. *Lancet* 1987; **2**: 709–711.

13. Grinstead WC, Francis MJ, Marks GF et al. Discontinuation of chronic diuretic therapy in stable congestive-heart-failure patients. *Circulation* 1992; **86**: 808.

14. Bayliss J, Norell M, Canepaanson R et al. Untreated heart-failure—clinical and neuroendocrine effects of introducing diuretics. *Br Heart J* 1987; **57**: 17–22.

15. Patterson JH, Adams KF, Applefeld MM, Corder CN, Masse BR. Oral torsemide in patients with chronic congestive-heart-failure—effects on body-weight, edema, and electrolyte excretion. *Pharmacotherapy* 1994; **14**: 514–521.

16. Sherman LG, Liang CS, Baumgardner S et al. Piretanide, a potent diuretic with potassium-sparing properties, for the treatment of congestive-heart-failure. *Clin Pharmacol Ther* 1986; **40**: 587–594.

17. Grinstead WC, Francis MJ, Marks GF et al. Discontinuation of chronic diuretic therapy in stable congestive-heart-failure secondary to coronary-artery disease or to idiopathic dilated cardiomyopathy. *Am J Cardiol* 1994; **73**: 881–886.

18. Remme WJ, Bodin F. Benzepril heart failure study. Is monotherapy with ACE inhibition preferable to diuretics in mild heart failure? A comparison of benazepril and hydrochlorothiazide. *J Am Coll Cardiol* 1996; **27**: 228A.

19. Cowley AJ, Stainer K, Wynne RD et al. Symptomatic assessment of patients with heart-failure—double-blind comparison of increasing doses of diuretics and captopril in moderate heart-failure. *Lancet* 1986; **2**: 770–772.

20. Lewis SJ, Roberts CJC. Double-blind comparison of high-dose bumetanide and half-dose bumetanide together with captopril in heart-failure. *Curr Ther Res Clin Exp* 1991; **50**: 3–13.

21. Francis GS, Siegel RM, Goldsmith SR et al. Acute vasoconstrictor response to intravenous furosemide in patients with chronic congestive heart-failure—activation of the neurohumoral axis. *Ann Int Med* 1985; **103**: 1–6.

22. Ikram H, Chan W, Espiner EA, Nicholls MG. Haemodynamic and hormone responses to acute and chronic furosemide therapy in chronic heart failure. *Clin Sci* 1980; **59**: 449.

23. Kubo SH, Clark M, Laragh JH et al. Identification of normal neurohormonal activity in mild congestive-heart-failure and stimulating effect of upright posture and diuretics. *Am J Cardiol* 1987; **60**: 1322–1328.

24. Francis GS, Benedict C, Johnstone DE et al. Comparison of neuroendocrine activation in patients with left-ventricular dysfunction with and without congestive-heart-failure—a substudy of the studies of left-ventricular dysfunction (Solvd). *Circulation* 1990; **82**: 1724–1729.

25. Wilcox CS, Mitch WE, Kelly RA et al. Response of the kidney to furosemide. 1. Effects of salt intake and renal compensation. *J Lab Clin Med* 1983; **102**: 450–458.

26. Gerlag PGG, Vanmeijel JJM. High-dose furosemide in the treatment of refractory congestive heart-failure. *Arch Int Med* 1988; **148**: 286–291.

27. Lahav M, Regev A, Raanani P, Theodor E. Intermittent administration of furosemide vs continuous infusion preceded by a loading dose for congestive-heart-failure. *Chest* 1992; **102**: 725–731.

28. Channer KS, Mclean KA, Lawsonmatthew P, Richardson M. Combination diuretic treatment in severe heart-failure—a randomized controlled trial. *Br Heart J* 1994; **71**: 146–150.

29. Agostini PG, Marenzi GD, Pepi M. Isolated ultrafiltration in moderate congestive heart failure. *J Am Coll Cardiol* 1993; **21**: 424.

30. Rubin J, Ball R. Continuous ambulatory peritoneal-dialysis as treatment of severe congestive-heart-failure in the face of chronic-renal-failure—report of 8 cases. *Arch Int Med* 1986; **146**: 1533–1535.

31. Inoue T, Sakai Y, Morooka S et al. Hemofiltration as treatment for patients with refractory heart-failure. *Clin Cardiol* 1992; **15**: 514–518.

32. Channavsin P, Seiwell R, Brater DC. Pharmacokinetic-dynamic analysis of the indomethacin–furosemide interaction in man. *J Pharmacol Exp Ther* 1980; **215**: 77.

33. Heerdink ER, Leufkens HG, Herings RMC et al. NSAIDs associated with increased risk of congestive heart failure in elderly patients taking diuretics. *Arch Int Med* 1998; **158**: 1108–1112.

34. Northridge DB, Currie PF, Newby DE et al. Placebo-controlled comparison of candoxatril, an orally active neutral endopeptidase inhibitor, and captopril in patients with chronic heart failure. *Eur J Heart Failure* 1999; **1**: 67–72.

Digoxin in chronic heart failure

Andrew Clark

6

Background

Although cardiac glycosides have been used for many thousands of years, William Withering described their clinical use in detail only in the 18th century.[1] Withering's source for his drug was the common foxglove, *Digitalis purpurea*, from which digitoxin is derived. Digoxin derives from *Digitalis lanata*. One of the richest doctors outside London, Withering has a foxglove carved on his memorial stone.

Digoxin is used for two distinct properties in the management of heart failure: it reduces the ventricular rate in patients with atrial fibrillation, and it has a positive inotropic effect. In Britain, it has primarily been used for the control of the ventricular response, but elsewhere, particularly in the United States, digoxin is prescribed much more widely. Despite this, it is only in recent years that randomized controlled trials of digoxin have been conducted.

Mechanism of action

Inotropic effects

Digoxin and the cardiac glycosides produce a positive

inotropic effect by inhibiting the cardiac sarcolemmal Na^+/K^+-ATPase (see *Figure 6.1*). Na^+/K^+-ATPase inhibition results in a rise in intracellular sodium. The sodium/calcium exchanger is largely driven by the gradient of sodium across the cell membrane. When the cell is depolarized, high intracellular sodium drives the exchanger with a resulting increase in intracellular calcium. When the cell is polarized, the increase in intracellular sodium induced by digoxin reduces the sodium gradient across the membrane, reducing the exchanger's activity and causing the extrusion of calcium.

The net consequence of digoxin administration is an increase in intracellular calcium available for myocyte contraction.

Electrophysiological effects

Digoxin has a vagotonic effect on cardiac electrophysiology with an increase in resting membrane potential, a reduction in automaticity and a reduction in conduction velocity, particularly through the atrioventricular node. The electrocardiogram often develops ST segment depression ('reversed tick') (Figure 6.2) in the lateral leads.

At toxic doses, digoxin can precipitate arrhythmias. This may be related to the accumulation of intracellular calcium and increased spontaneous electrical activity.

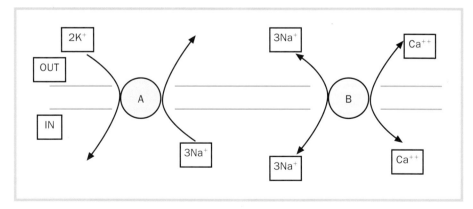

Figure 6.1
Selected ion channels and pumps involved in the positive inotropic effect of digoxin. A is the 'sodium pump' Na^+/K^+-ATPase). B is the sodium/calcium exchanger. When the cell is polarized, sodium entering the cell causes calcium to leave. When the cell is depolarized, the higher intracellular sodium drives the exchanger in the opposite direction. See text for details

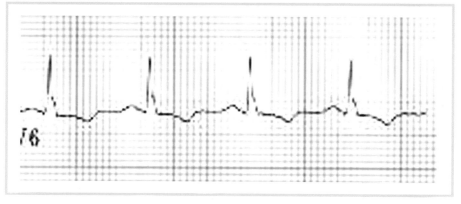

Figure 6.2
Electrocardiographic recording of lead V6. The patient is in sinus rhythm and receiving digoxin. The ST depression shows the 'reversed tick' abnormality.

Autonomic effects

Digoxin has complex effects on the autonomic nervous system. These include an increase in sympathetic outflow when administered acutely. In chronic heart failure, digoxin results in suppression of plasma noradrenaline (norepinephrine).[2,3] Digoxin also appears to reduce the sympathetic response to exercise.[2] These changes are seen in conjunction with a return of the baroreflex sensitivity towards normal.[4,5]

Effects on the renin-angiotensin-aldosterone system

There is evidence that digoxin reduces both plasma renin activity and plasma aldosterone concentration in heart failure.[6]

Digoxin in sinus rhythm: trial evidence

Despite the duration of digoxin's use in clinical practice, until recently there have been few data to support its use in heart failure, particularly in patients with sinus rhythm. Other positive inotropic agents tested in randomized studies have been uniformly disappointing with increases in mortality with, for example, milrinone,[7] vesnarinone[8] and xamoterol.[9] Some studies have suggested that digoxin can increase mortality when used after myocardial infarction.[10,11]

Small trials in the 1980s[12,13] suggested that digoxin exerted a beneficial effect, but these were small, and often complicated by a crossover design. Half the patients would therefore be *withdrawing* from digoxin, which may not be the same as never receiving it in the first place. The Captopril–Digoxin trial[14] was a much larger study (300 patients, *Table 6.1*). The patients were randomized to digoxin, captopril or placebo. In the digoxin group, there was an improvement in left ventricular ejection fraction not seen in the captopril group. There were no effects on exercise capacity or symptoms. However, 65% of the patients had been on long-term digoxin before the trial; the patients had mild heart failure only. Interestingly, the number of ventricular premature beats decreased by 45% in the captopril group and increased by 4% in the digoxin group.

The Captopril and Digoxin study[15] randomized 63 patients to captopril, 66 to digoxin and 67 to placebo. The patients had class II–III heart failure. After a year, digoxin resulted in an improvement in general well-being and symptom score, but cardiovascular events during follow-up were lower in the captopril group than in those on placebo and digoxin.

The German–Austrian xamoterol study[16] randomized patients to digoxin, xamoterol or placebo. There was no change in exercise capacity, but digoxin did result in improvements in symptoms. Xamoterol improved exercise capacity. However, the level of left ventricular function is not reported in the study, and only a quarter of the patients

were taking a diuretic, suggesting very mild heart failure.

DiBianco et al[17] reported the results of a comparison of milrinone, digoxin, the combination of the two and placebo in 230 patients with an ejection fraction of 25%. At 3 months, digoxin led to an improvement in left ventricular ejection fraction and exercise capacity compared with milrinone. On the face of it, this is a curious result, as the digoxin limb was a *continuation* of digoxin that the patients were all taking at the outset of the study, not a new initiation.

The DIMT study[17] compared digoxin (n = 55) with ibopamine (n = 53) or placebo (n = 53). At 6 months' follow up, the digoxin group had a greater exercise capacity than the placebo group. Further, there were benefits in neurohormonal activation with lower noradrenaline and renin in the digoxin-treated patients.

The studies discussed so far do not lead to a satisfactory understanding of the role of digoxin. By present standards, they were small studies, and in some the patient groups were imperfectly characterized. The studies were designed as comparative studies between digoxin and another agent, and were conducted against background treatment that would now be considered inadequate, particularly as regards angiotensin converting enzyme (ACE) inhibitors.

The PROVED[18] and RADIANCE[19] studies were randomized, placebo-controlled

Table 6.1
Trials of digoxin in patients with heart failure in sinus rhythm

Trial	Year	n	Time (weeks)	NYHA	LVEF (%)	Study drug	Withdrawal	End-points	Results (Dig vs. placebo)
Captopril–digoxin[14]	1988	300	24	II–III	26	Dig vs. capto vs. placebo	Yes	LVEF Exercise Symptoms	↑15% No change No change
German–Austrian[16]	1988	433	12	II, 71%*	?	Dig vs. xamoterol vs. placebo	Yes	Exercise Symptoms	Small benefit No change
DiBianco et al[17]	1989	230	12	III, >60%	25	Dig vs. milrinone vs. placebo vs. both	Yes	LVEF Exercise	↑1.7%† ↑14%
Just et al[15]	1993	222	52	II–III	50	Dig vs. capto vs. placebo	Yes	Exercise Symptoms	No change Small benefit
Ibopamine[18]	1993	161	26	II, 80%	28	Dig vs. ibopamine vs. placebo	Yes	Events Exercise Noradrenaline	No change† Increase Decrease
PROVED[19]	1993	88	12	II, >80%	28	Dig vs. placebo	Yes	Exercise Treatment failure	Dig better Less than placebo
RADIANCE[20]	1993	178	12	II, >70%	27	Dig vs. placebo	Yes	LVEF Exercise Treatment failure LVEF	Small increase Dig better Less than placebo Less than placebo

NYHA, New York Heart Association classification of symptoms in heart failure; LVEF, left ventricular ejection fraction; Dig, digoxin; capto, captopril.
*Only 25% were receiving diuretic.
†This was digoxin continuation, not new treatment.
‡Events lower in captopril group.

studies of digoxin *withdrawal* against a background of treatment with diuretics alone (PROVED) or diuretics plus ACE inhibitors (RADIANCE). The major end-points were incidence of treatment failure, treadmill exercise time and 6-minute walk test distance. In addition, the investigators considered quality of life and measurements of left ventricular function. Follow-up was 12 weeks.

The PROVED study was stopped prematurely, owing to low recruitment (ACE inhibitors were widely used), and only 88 patients were randomized. Nevertheless, there was a fall in treadmill time in the placebo group and an increase in treatment failure. There were no differences in quality of life scores or in left ventricular ejection fraction.

In RADIANCE, 93 patients received placebo, and 85 digoxin. Treadmill time deteriorated in the placebo group, and there was a much greater incidence of treatment failure on placebo. Quality of life deteriorated less in the digoxin group, as did left ventricular ejection fraction.

PROVED and RADIANCE provoked much debate. Both studies were very short term, and not powered to detect effects on mortality. Crucially, they were both withdrawal studies. This testifies to the difficulties of trying to identify enough patients with heart failure who are not taking digoxin, particularly in America. Testing withdrawal of a drug against its continuation is *not* the same as testing the drug and

placebo. If digoxin exerts a positive inotropic effect, it might well improve heart failure but at the same time be toxic (perhaps owing to slow accumulation of intracellular calcium). Abrupt withdrawal would result in deterioration as inotropic support is removed and the toxic effect revealed.

The DIG trial[21] was designed to address this issue. At the time, it was the largest randomized trial in heart failure; 3397 patients were randomized to digoxin and 3403 to placebo. The majority of patients were in NYHA class II and III heart failure, and the average left ventricular ejection fraction was 28%. Nearly 95% were receiving ACE inhibitors at entry, and all were in sinus rhythm; 44% were receiving digoxin at study entry. There was no wash-out period before randomization, so that any withdrawal effect would be noted. Follow-up was for an average of 37 months, with a primary end-point of all-cause mortality. There was a smaller ancillary trial for patients with heart failure and a normal ejection fraction (492 digoxin, 496 placebo).

There was no difference between the two groups in all-cause mortality, which was approximately 35% in both groups (*Figure 6.3*). Interestingly, there was an increase in sudden death in the digoxin group, but this was offset by a reduction in deaths due to worsening heart failure.

There was a reduction in the combined end-point of death or hospitalization for worsening heart failure. From the patients'

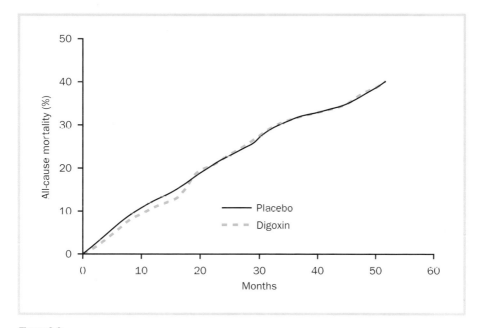

Figure 6.3
The principle results of the DIG trial. Redrawn, with permission, from reference 20

perspective, however, the cause of admission is less important than the fact of admission. There was a significant reduction in all cause admission, but this was a smaller effect than on heart failure admission. The results in the ancillary trial (of heart failure with normal ejection fraction) were similar, although mortality was lower than for the main trial at 23%.

DIG does not provide the definitive answer to the question of digoxin use in sinus rhythm. Although the dose was titrated in the trial to a target digoxin level, there was a three-fold variation in achieved level (0.5–2.0 ng/ml). Whether higher levels confer additional benefit, or indeed harm, is not clear.

Digoxin in atrial fibrillation

Chronic heart failure and atrial fibrillation are both common, and they commonly coexist. Atrial fibrillation is more common with increasing severity of heart failure, being seen in around 10% of patients with mild to moderate heart failure, rising to around 50% in class IV heart failure.[22]

Digoxin is almost universally prescribed to control the ventricular rate of patients with atrial fibrillation and chronic heart failure. Concerns about the safety of other potential rate-controlling agents in heart failure (the negative inotropic effects of verapamil and diltiazem; proarrhythmic effects of class I agents; widespread side-effects of amiodarone) have meant that this role for digoxin has not been challenged. However, the new evidence supporting the role of β-adrenoceptor antagonists in heart failure mean that here, too, the role of digoxin may be limited.

Digoxin does not increase the chances of a return to sinus rhythm in acute atrial fibrillation,[23] and whilst it certainly does reduce the resting ventricular rate in lone atrial fibrillation, it does not control the heart rate during exercise[24] and may not do so in more severe heart failure.[25] There are, as yet, no published data comparing digoxin and β-blockade, or indeed their combination, in atrial fibrillation in chronic heart failure. The CAFÉ study[26] has addressed this question explicitly, and the results should be available soon.

Clinical use of digoxin

What is the role for digoxin in patients with chronic heart failure? As advances in

therapeutics are made, older drugs may no longer be the best. With the introduction of loop diuretics, then successively vasodilators and ACE inhibitors and now β-blockers, the clinical role for digoxin has gradually become superseded. It seems likely that digoxin will be used less and less.

At present, the primary indication for digoxin in sinus rhythm is for symptomatic benefit. In practical terms, this means that patients with class III or IV symptoms, particularly patients with a resting tachycardia and with a third heart sound, are likely to gain most benefit.

In patients with atrial fibrillation, digoxin will continue to be widely used for ventricular rate control. The CAFÉ study should answer the question as to whether β-blockade may be better in this regard. In very sick patients in whom β-blockers cannot be used, digoxin will still have a role.

Dosing

Digoxin has a relatively narrow therapeutic window, and needs to be used with some caution. The half-life is up to 48 hours. The dose of digoxin used is often inappropriately low. An adult male of normal size with normal renal function will need 250 µg daily, with some patients needing more. A dose of 62.5 µg is rarely necessary. Plasma digoxin levels serve as a guide to treatment (although toxicity can occur in the therapeutic range).

Blood should be taken at least 6 hours following oral administration.

Side-effects

Particular care needs to be taken to prevent hypokalaemia, as this increases the toxic effects. Renal impairment, so common in heart failure, will also enhance the digoxin effect. Anorexia and nausea are the commonest symptoms of excess digoxin, and vomiting and diarrhoea my occur. Visual disturbance is less frequent, and a few patients describe xanthopsia, where objects appear yellow.

The risk of arrhythmia, both bradycardia and tachycardia, is the greatest concern with digoxin use. If a patient describes worsening palpitations or dizzy turns, these must be taken very seriously. In a life-threatening situation, Digibind® (digoxin-specific antibody fragments) can be used to reduce the toxic effects of digoxin.

References

1. Withering W. An account of the foxglove and some of its medical uses, with practical remarks on dropsy and other diseases. In: Willius FA, Keys TE (eds). *Classics of Cardiology*. Baltimore: Dover Publications, 1941: 231.

2. Ribner HS, Plucinski DA, Hseieh AM et al. Acute effects of digoxin on total systemic vascular resistance in congestive heart failure due to dilated cardiomyopathy. *Am J Cardiol* 1985; **56:** 896–904.

3. Covit AB, Schaer GI, Sealey JE et al. Suppression of the renin–angiotensin system by intravenous digoxin in chronic congestive heart failure. *Am J Med* 1983; **75:** 445–447.

4. Ferguson DW. Baroreflex-mediated circulatory control in human heart failure. *Heart Failure* 1990; **6:** 3–11.

5. Ferguson DW, Berg WJ, Saunders JS et al. Sympathoinhibitory responses to digitalis glycosides in heart failure patients. *Circulation* 1989; **80:** 65–77.

6. Covit AB, Schaer GL, Sealey JE et al. Suppression of the renin-angiotensin system by intravenous digoxin in chronic congestive heart failure. *Am J Med* 1983; **75:** 445–447.

7. Packer M, Carver JR, Rodeheffer RJ et al., for the PROMISE Study Research Group. Effect of oral milrinone on mortality in severe chronic heart failure. *N Engl J Med* 1991; **325:** 1468–1475.

8. Cohn JN, Goldstein SO, Greenberg BH et al. A dose-dependent increase in mortality with vesnarinone among patients with severe heart failure. *N Engl J Med* 1998; **339:** 1810–1816.

9. The Xamoterol in Severe Heart Failure Study Group. Xamoterol in severe heart failure. *Lancet* 1990; **336:** 1–6.

10. Moss AJ, Davis HT, Conard DL et al. Digitalis-associated cardiac mortality after myocardial infarction. *Circulation* 1981; **64:** 1150–1156.

11. Bigger JT Jr, Fleiss JL, Rolnitzky LM et al. Effect of digitalis treatment on survival after acute myocardial infarction. *Am J Cardiol* 1985; **55:** 623–630.

12. Fleg JL, Gottlieb SH, Lakatta EG. Is digoxin really important in treatment of compensated

heart failure? A placebo-controlled crossover study in patients with sinus rhythm. *Am J Med* 1982; **73**: 244–250.

13. Lee DC, Johnson RA, Bingham JB et al. Heart failure in outpatients: a randomized trial of digoxin versus placebo. *N Engl J Med* 1982; **306**: 699–705.

14. The Captopril–Digoxin Multicenter Research Group. Comparative effects of therapy with captopril and digoxin in patients with mild to moderate heart failure. *J Am Med Assoc* 1988; **259**: 539–544.

15. Just H, Drexler H, Taylor SH et al. Captopril versus digoxin in patients with coronary artery disease and mild heart failure. A prospective, double-blind, placebo-controlled multicenter study. The CADS Study Group. *Herz* 1993; **18 (Suppl 1)**: 436–443.

16. The German and Austrian Xamoterol Study Group. Double-blind placebo-controlled comparison of digoxin and xamoterol in chronic heart failure. *Lancet* 1988; **1**: 489–493.

17. DiBianco R, Shabetai R, Kostuk W et al. Comparison of oral milrinone, digoxin, and their combination in the treatment of patients with chronic heart failure. *N Engl J Med* 1989; **320**: 677–683.

18. van Veldhuisen DJ, Man in 't Veld AJ, Dunselman PH et al. Double-blind placebo-controlled study of ibopamine and digoxin in patients with mild to moderate heart failure: results of the Dutch Ibopamine Multicenter Trial (DIMT). *J Am Coll Cardiol* 1993; **22**: 1564–1573.

19. Uretsky BF, Young JB, Shahidi FE et al. Randomized study assessing the effect of digoxin withdrawal in patients with mild to moderate chronic congestive heart failure: results of the PROVED trial. PROVED Investigative Group. *J Am Coll Cardiol* 1993; **22**: 955–962.

20. Packer M, Gheorghiade M, Young JB et al. Withdrawal of digoxin from patients with chronic heart failure treated with angiotensin-converting-enzyme inhibitors. RADIANCE Study. *N Engl J Med* 1993; **329**: 1–7.

21. The Digitalis Investigation Group. The effect of digoxin on mortality and mortidity in patients with heart failure *N Engl J Med* 1997; **336**: 525–533.

22. The CONSENSUS trial study group. Effects of enalapril on mortality in severe congestive heart failure: results of the Cooperative North Scandinavian Enalapril Survival Study (CONSENSUS). *N Engl J Med* 1987; **316**: 1429–1435.

23. Hou ZY, Chang MS, Chen CY et al. Acute treatment of recent-onset atrial fibrillation and flutter with a tailored dosing regimen of intravenous amiodarone. A randomized, digoxin-controlled study. *Eur Heart J* 1995; **16**: 521–528.

24. Beasley R, Smith DA, McHaffie DJ. Exercise heart rates at different serum digoxin concentrations in patients with atrial fibrillation. *Br Med J* 1985; **290**: 9–11.

25. Goldman S, Probst P, Selzer A, Cohn K. Inefficacy of 'therapeutic' serum levels of digoxin in controlling the ventricular rate in atrial fibrillation. *Am J Cardiol* 1975; **35**: 651–655.

26. McGowan J, Cleland JGF. Carvedilol in heart failure. Trials in progress. *Heart Fail Rev* 1999; **4**: 89–95.

Treatment: inhibitors of the renin–angiotensin-aldosterone system

Neal Padmanabhan

7

This chapter discusses the use of inhibitors of the renin–angiotensin-aldosterone system (RAAS) in the treatment of chronic heart failure. Because most of the available evidence refers to left ventricular systolic dysfunction, this will be considered here. Treatment of chronic heart failure has two main aims: to alleviate symptoms and to improve prognosis. A number of large clinical trials have shown that inhibitors of the RAAS, mainly angiotensin converting enzyme (ACE) inhibitors, improve symptoms, increase exercise capacity, reduce hospitalization and, perhaps most importantly, improve survival in patient with heart failure. Therefore, these form the mainstay of the pharmacological treatment of all grades of chronic heart failure and, in the absence of specific contraindications, their use is now considered mandatory. This chapter discusses the rationale for their use, summarizes the evidence for their efficacy, describes guidelines for their initiation and considers areas in which therapy based on the inhibition of the RAAS can be improved.

Physiology and pathophysiology of the renin–angiotensin-aldosterone system in chronic heart failure

The RAAS is an enzyme cascade that generates the octapeptide angiotensin II.[1] *Figure 7.1* details the principal steps in the cascade and indicates the points at which it can be inhibited. Angiotensin II has long been known to mediate vasoconstriction, promote sodium retention and stimulate aldosterone release. Aldosterone may also be considered an effector hormone of the RAAS.[2] Angiotensin II promotes sodium and water retention and is crucial in the regulation of peripheral resistance. It has been shown to promote the proliferation of a variety of cell types, including vascular smooth muscle cells, fibroblasts and mesangial cells, and to stimulate the deposition of extracellular matrix in a number of tissues, including the heart.[3–5] These effects are frequently mediated in a paracrine fashion through the action of a number of cytokines and growth factors.[6,7] The components of the RAAS are found in tissues as well as the circulation. However, the relative importance of the systemic and tissue systems is not yet clear.

Chronic heart failure is associated with neurohormonal dysfunction and activation of the RAAS.[8] Activation of the RAAS (and other neurohormonal systems) seems to have evolved as a response to a fall in tissue perfusion pressure. In evolutionary terms this was presumably a response to acute blood loss of salt and water depletion. However, in heart failure, neurohormonal activation is a maladaptive response that contributes to the progression of chronic heart failure through a variety of mechanisms.[9] The RAAS increases cardiac preload and afterload by salt and water retention and vasoconstriction, and also contributes to cardiac remodelling, with fibrosis and, possibly, myocyte apoptosis.[10] Endothelial dysfunction and peripheral muscle abnormalities together with both renal and pulmonary homeostatic abnormalities are related to neurohormonal activation. Thus, while neurohormonal activation may be beneficial acutely in preserving tissue perfusion, it may then be deleterious. The logical conclusion from this hypothesis is that treatments which reduce neurohormonal activation may not only improve symptoms, but also slow the progression of the syndrome. This forms the physiological basis for inhibition of the RAAS.

Inhibitors of the renin–angiotensin-aldosterone system in clinical practice

The RAAS can be inhibited at a number of points. As early studies found the conversion of angiotensinogen to angiotensin I by renin to be the rate-limiting step, great efforts have been made to develop inhibitors of this

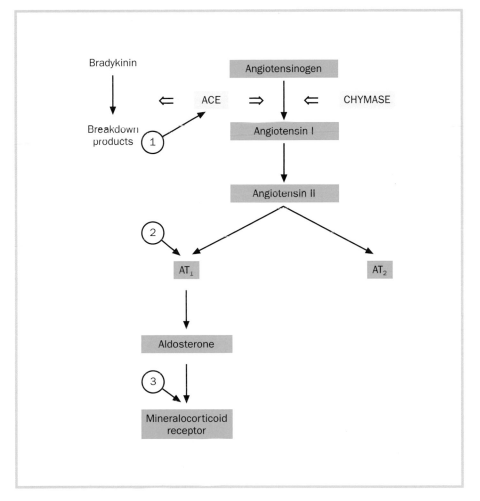

Figure 7.1
The enzyme cascade of the renin–angiotensin system. Angiotensinogen in the circulation is converted to angiotensin I by the action of renin. Renin is released from the maccula densa of the kidney in response to a fall in perfusion pressure and sympathetic nervous system activation. In turn, angiotensin I is converted to angiotensin II by angiotensin converting enzyme (ACE). Additional enzymes, such as chymase, can mediate this step. Angiotensin II mediates its effects through receptors, AT_1 and AT_2. AT_1 is responsible for vasoconstriction and for aldosterone release.

enzyme. However, no orally available agents have become available, so in practice the RAAS may be inhibited by ACE inhibitors or angiotensin II type 1 receptor (AT$_1$) antagonists. Aldosterone antagonists, such as spironolactone, can also be considered to be inhibitors of the RAAS.

Treatment of chronic heart failure using angiotensin converting enzyme inhibitors

The use of ACE inhibitors in chronic heart failure has been studied in a number of large randomized controlled studies, with consistently encouraging results. The results of these studies are summarized in *Table 7.1*.

In the CONSENSUS I the effect of the addition of enalapril to conventional therapy was studied in 253 patients with severe (NYHA class IV) chronic heart failure.[11] This trial was discontinued early because of the marked benefit of ACE inhibitor treatment. Not only was there a significant symptomatic improvement, but mortality was reduced by 40% at 6 months and 31% at 1 year. This was accompanied by an improvement in the NYHA classification and less need for additional medication. At the end of the study there were 135 survivors, 58 in the placebo group and 77 in the enalapril group. Ten-year follow-up data are now available from this study.[12] At 10 years there were only five survivors, all in the enalapril group. The benefit of enalapril during the double-blind period was clearly carried over beyond the end of the trial, since there was a lag of 6–12 months before the merging of the survival curves of those who received the drug during the trial and those who started open-label

Table 7.1
Major trials with angiotensin converting enzyme inhibitors in chronic heart failure

Study	No. of patients	LVEF (%)	Study drug	Mortality (%) (drug:control)	p Value
CONSENSUS I	253	—	Enalapril	39:54	0.003
SOLVD Treatment	2569	25	Enalapril	35.2:39.7	0.003
SOLVD Prevention	4228	28	Enalapril	14.8:15.8	0.3
Ve HeFT II	804	29	Enalapril	32.8:38.2	0.08

LVEF, left ventricular ejection fraction

medication afterwards. Those patients who did not receive open-label enalapril at the conclusion of the double-blind period had a considerably higher mortality compared to those who did.

The effect of ACE inhibition in mild to moderate chronic heart failure was studied in a much larger trial, SOLVD. This study had two arms. The treatment trial randomized patients with symptomatic mild to moderate chronic heart failure and ejection fractions of <35% (n = 2569) to enalapril versus conventional therapy. The prevention trial studied patients with asymptomatic low ejection fractions (again <35%; n = 4228), to assess the ability of enalapril to prevent progression of the syndrome.[13,14] After a mean follow-up of 41.1 months the mortality of patients in the treatment trial was reduced by 16%, mostly accounted for by a reduction in progressive heart failure. There was also a significant reduction of 40% in the rate of hospitalization, when the combined end-point of death or hospitalization at 1 year was considered. In the prevention arm of the study a similar pattern was observed, although the effect of enalapril was less marked. These studies confirmed not only that treatment with an ACE inhibitor reduced mortality in chronic heart failure, but that this was largely achieved by a reduction in deaths from progressive heart failure, and that benefit was also obtained in asymptomatic patients. In fact, because patients in the placebo group

received new therapies, or increased doses of existing drugs, the analysis probably underestimated the degree of benefit achieved with enalapril. Based on the results of SOLVD, treating 1000 patients with enalapril for 3 years would prevent 50 deaths and 350 hospitalizations.

The first Veterans Administration trial, V-HeFT I, of vasodilator therapy with hydralazine and isosorbide dinitrate (ISDN) versus placebo in chronic heart failure showed a treatment benefit.[15] Accordingly a second trial, V-HeFT II, was undertaken to compare hydralazine plus ISDN with ACE inhibitors. The prognosis was better in those given enalapril, with a reduction in mortality of 11.1% at the end of the follow-up period.[16] Interestingly, greater benefit was seen in the enalapril-treated group despite a lack of improvement in exercise capacity, which increased during the first 6 months of hydralazine plus ISDN treatment. This suggests that the two forms of therapy did not have the same mode of action and that enalapril conferred additional benefit beyond its role as a vasodilator.

A meta-analysis of the use of ACE inhibitors in the treatment of chronic heart failure[17] confirmed the results of individual studies, showing a reduction in overall mortality of 23% and a reduction in combined mortality and hospitalization for chronic heart failure of 35%. The effect was observed with several different ACE inhibitors, although data were largely for enalapril, captopril, ramipril and lisinopril. The greatest benefit was seen in those with the lowest ejection fractions, and after 3 months of therapy, but additional benefit was observed with prolonged treatment. The reduction in mortality was primarily due to fewer deaths from progressive heart failure.

The majority of patients in these landmark trials had chronic heart failure due to ischaemic heart disease (>70% of patients in CONSENSUS). This raises the question of whether treatment with ACE inhibitors in patients with left ventricular dysfunction early after myocardial infarction (MI) might be of benefit by reducing the progression to severe chronic heart failure. This has also been extensively studied.

Angiotensin converting enzyme inhibition after myocardial infarction

The results of the major studies of the use of ACE inhibitors in the post-MI period are summarized in *Table 7.2.*

In the SAVE trial 2231 patients with an ejection fraction of <40%, as identified by radionuclide ventriculography, were assigned to captopril or placebo from 3 to 16 days post-MI.[18] Those who received captopril had a reduction in the risk of death of 19% compared to those who received placebo. Hospitalization for chronic heart failure was reduced by 22% and the risk of recurrent MI

by 25%. During the trial, 13% of patients converted to open-label captopril, owing to the development of overt chronic heart failure. The development of overt heart failure was associated with an increased mortality; however, those randomized to captopril were less likely to require open-label treatment and were less likely to die once they did.

The TRACE trial studied the effect of treatment with trandolapril compared to placebo in 2606 patients with left ventricular systolic dysfunction, as defined by echocardiographically determined ejection fraction of <35%, 3 to 7 days post-MI.[19] Again, there was a reduction of the risk of death and of progression to severe heart failure, by 22% and 29%, respectively.

The AIRE trial differed from SAVE and TRACE in that eligibility was determined by the presence of clinical evidence of heart failure, rather than depending on an assessment of ejection fraction. In this study, treatment with ramipril was associated with a reduction in mortality of 27%.[20] Despite the fact that there was no pre-randomization run-in period and that, compared to SAVE and TRACE, patients were relatively unselected, ramipril was well tolerated and the clinical benefit was apparent early.

The results of the three trials described above should be contrasted with the results of the CONSENSUS II trial, in which treatment with enalapril was instituted within 24 hours of acute MI, with no assessment of left

Table 7.2
Major trials using angiotensin converting enzyme inhibitors in post-myocardial infarction left ventricular dysfunction

Study	No. of patients	LVEF (%)	Study drug	Mortality (%) (drug:control)	p Value
AIRE	2006	—	Ramipril	17:23	0.002
TRACE	1749	30	Trandolapril	34.7:42.3	0.001
SAVE	2231	31	Captopril	20:25	0.019

LVEF, left ventricular ejection fraction

ventricular function.[21] This trial was terminated early because of an increased mortality in the enalapril-treated group at 6 months. Taken together with the results of the much larger ISIS 4 and GISSI 3 trials, which did show a small benefit following treatment (with captopril and lisinopril, respectively) in unselected patients immediately post-MI, it would appear that the benefit of ACE inhibitor therapy in this situation is greatest in those with left ventricular dysfunction.[22,23]

In the light of the evidence above, it is therefore recommended that all patients with chronic heart failure due to left ventricular systolic dysfunction should receive an ACE inhibitor, unless there is a specific contraindication. This includes patients rendered asymptomatic with diuretic therapy.

Guidelines for the initiation of angiotensin converting enzyme inhibitor therapy in chronic heart failure

Despite the evidence that treatment with an ACE inhibitor reduces symptoms and improves mortality in patients with chronic heart failure, studies consistently report that these drugs are underprescribed. This may reflect concerns over their safety. Side-effects of ACE inhibitor therapy include symptomatic hypotension, renal impairment, hyperkalaemia, cough and other more idiosyncratic reactions such as rash and angio-oedema. Hypotension and renal impairment are more likely in patients whose blood pressure and glomerular filtration are renin-dependent, such as diuretic-treated patients who are sodium depleted. Hyperkalaemia is made more likely by the presence of pre-existing renal disease and concomitant therapy with 'potassium-sparing' diuretics. In the SOLVD study there was a significant increase in symptoms attributable to hypotension in the active group, but there was no significant difference in the proportion of patients taking their assigned medication at the end of the trial.[15] Similarly, in CONSENSUS I symptomatic hypotension was observed initially and led to a change in the titration protocol, with a slower escalation of dose in those considered to be at high risk (e.g. those with serum sodium levels of <130 mmol/l, or creatinine >150 μmol/l).[13] A retrospective analysis of the data from CONSENSUS I showed that, in enalapril-treated patients, there was an average increase in creatinine of 10–15% within 3 weeks, but that this did not increase thereafter.[24] In 24% of patients creatinine actually fell, probably because of an improvement in renal perfusion. Serum creatinine doubled in 11% of enalapril-treated patients (compared to 3% in patients on placebo). Multivariate analysis suggested that the strongest predictor of an abnormal increase in creatinine was hypotension and that this was itself predicted by a prior reduction in glomerular filtration rate.

The evidence suggests that ACE inhibitor therapy is generally safe, but caution should be exercised in patients in whom the RAAS is likely to be activated prior to commencement of treatment. An approach to initiation of therapy is given in *Figure 7.2*. Treatment should start with a low dose, e.g. captopril 6.25 mg thrice daily, or enalapril 5 mg twice daily, and be titrated upwards to the maximum tolerated dose over a period of days to weeks. If symptomatic hypotension occurs, or there is evidence of organ hypoperfusion, other hypotensive agents should be stopped unless specifically required. Patients at high risk of hypotension, such as those receiving high doses of diuretics, should receive a test dose of captopril 6.25 mg before commencing therapy with a long-acting drug. However, it is best, where possible, to reduce the diuretic dose prior to initiation of therapy. Potassium-sparing diuretics (except spironolactone) should be discontinued.

Choice and dose of angiotensin converting enzyme inhibitor

It is likely that the benefits of ACE inhibitors represent a class-effect, thus the choice of drug may be of subsidiary importance. Any of the drugs with proven benefit are acceptable. The greatest experience is probably with enalapril, ramipril, lisinopril and trandolapril. The target dose should be that which was shown to be beneficial in a clinical trial. Suggested doses are shown in *Table 7.3*. The use of these larger doses is supported by the ATLAS trial which showed a greater reduction in combined mortidity and mortality with high dose (32.5–35 mg) compared to low dose (2.5–5 mg) lisinopril.[25]

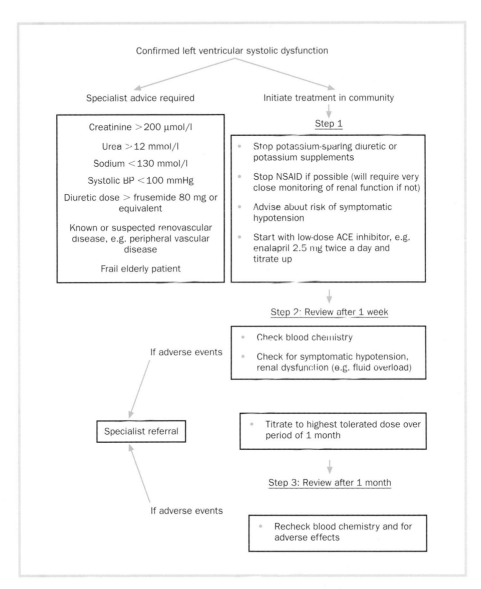

Figure 7.2
Guidelines for the initiation of angiotensin converting enzyme (ACE) inhibitors in chronic heart failure (adapted from the SIGN guidelines for the treatment of chronic heart failure).

Table 7.3
Target doses of angiotensin converting enzyme (ACE) inhibitors based on studies of heart failure and post-infarction left ventricular dysfunction (taken from the SIGN guidelines for the treatment of chronic heart failure).

ACE inhibitor	Dose	Dosing schedule
Captopril	50–100 mg	Thrice daily
Enalapril	10–20 mg	Twice daily
Ramipril	5 mg	Twice daily
Trandolapril	4 mg	Once daily
Lisinopril	30–35 mg	Once daily

Angiotensin II receptor antagonists

Although treatment with an ACE inhibitor undeniably improves outcome in patients with chronic heart failure, their prognosis remains poor. In CONSENSUS I mortality at 1 year was 36% and in Ve HeFT II the 4-year cumulative mortality was 41%, despite enalapril therapy.[13,16] There remains, therefore, considerable scope for improvement. Angiotensin II type I receptor antagonists have attracted attention for a number of reasons.

There is evidence that treatment with ACE inhibitors does not completely suppress the RAAS. Thus, while angiotensin II levels initially fall, long-term suppression is not observed with ACE inhibitor therapy.[26] Angiotensin II levels may even rebound to their previous (elevated) levels and this has been correlated with deterioration in left ventricular function.[27] There are a number of

reasons for this phenomenon. ACE is not the rate-limiting step in the RAAS. Thus, following administration of an ACE inhibitor, there will be an increase in renin and angiotensin I concentrations due to interruption of feedback. As the plasma levels of the inhibitor fall towards the end of a dosing interval, angiotensin II will therefore increase, driven by the high precursor levels. This could explain the flat dose–response curve on blood pressure observed with ACE inhibitors.[28] In addition, there is evidence that alternative non-ACE pathways exist for the generation of angiotensin II, such as human chymase.[29] In chronically ACE-inhibited patients, angiotensin I may be shunted through these pathways, accounting for the escape of angiotensin II.

By directly blocking the receptor responsible for most of the biological actions of angiotensin II, these receptor antagonists may circumvent those problems. In addition, they have fewer side-effects, especially in that cough is not observed. Hence, receptor antagonists are a potential alternative to ACE inhibitors in the treatment of chronic heart failure. While theoretically attractive the angiotensin II type I receptor antagonists have to be tested in clinical trials.

ELITE II was therefore mounted,[30] which was designed to compare the effect of losartan and captopril on patient survival in chronic heart failure. A total of 3152 patients with NYHA class II-IV heart failure were randomly assigned to losartan (dose titrated to 50 mg daily) or captopril (50 mg thrice daily). The primary end-point was all-cause mortality. The estimated annual mortality was 11.7% in losartan-treated patients, and 10.4% in captopril-treated patients. The risk of sudden death was 9.0% in losartan treated patients, and 7.3% in captopril-treated patients. These differences were not significant. ACE inhibitors should continue to be the treatment of choice in chronic heart failure. Other ongoing trials, ValHeFT and CHARM are testing the place of angiotensin II type I receptor antagonists.[31,32]

Combined angiotensin inhibitor and receptor antagonist therapy

Another strategy that follows from the failure of ACE inhibitors to produce complete suppression of angiotensin II levels is to combine ACE inhibitors and receptor antagonists. This strategy has been tested in short-term studies on blood pressure, in which the combination had been found to be more effective than either drug alone and also more effective than increasing the dose of the ACE inhibitor.[33] In addition to a more complete suppression of the RAAS, this approach also has the theoretical advantage of maintaining the potentiation of bradykinin seen with ACE inhibitors. Since bradykinin is partly responsible for the short-term hypotensive effect of ACE inhibitors, it is even possible that kinins play a significant role in the long-term effects of ACE inhibitors in chronic heart failure.[34] While one small study suggests combination ACE inhibitor angiotensin II type I receptor antagonist therapy improves symptoms and exercise tolerance, the result of the ValHeFT and CHARM trials are awaited before this therapeutic approach can be supported.[35]

Aldosterone antagonism: spironolactone

Aldosterone is a mineralocorticoid hormone for which angiotensin II is the principal physiological regulator. Aldosterone levels are elevated in chronic heart failure and are not fully suppressed by ACE inhibitors. The hormone has a number of adverse effects in chronic heart failure. It acts on the distal tubules of the kidney to promote sodium and water resorption and has growth-promoting properties that are implicated in myocardial remodelling. Aldosterone may also have pro-arrhythmic effects through a number of mechanisms, such as myocardial fibrosis, K^+ depletion and sympathetic nervous system activation. Spironolactone antagonizes aldosterone.

RALES was a placebo-controlled study of spironolactone in 1663 patients with severe (NHYA class III-IV) chronic heart failure.[36] It showed a 30% reduction of the risk of death and hospitalization for cardiac causes and an improvement in the NYHA class in patients who received spironolactone. Patients were already on conventional treatment with ACE inhibitors, diuretic and, where indicated, digoxin. To be eligible for the study renal function had to be relatively well preserved (creatinine ≤221 μmol/l). Contrary to expectations, hyperkalaemia was not a serious problem, although 10% of patients treated with spironolactone withdrew because of gynaecomastia or breast pain. On the basis of this study spironolactone should be commenced in patients with severe chronic heart failure who have good renal function. Appropriate monitoring of serum K^+ should be performed.

Other possible therapeutic strategies: combined angiotensin converting enzyme inhibitors and neutral endopeptidase inhibition

Neutral endopeptidase (NEP) cleaves and inactivates natriuretic peptides. These peptides, of which atrial natriuretic peptide (ANP) was the first to be identified, are thought to be cardioprotective, since they promote sodium excretion, cause vasodilatation, suppress the RAAS and have antiproliferative properties. Their plasma concentrations are increased by NEP inhibition. 'Vasopeptidase inhibitors' combine in a single molecule the ability to inhibit ACE and NEP. The first such drug to reach clinical trails was omapatrilat. Animal studies suggested that this drug was more effective than ACE inhibition alone in improving haemodynamic abnormalities in chronic heart failure.[37] In one preliminary clinical study omapatrilat seemed to improve a CHF composite end-point more than lisinopril.[38]

A note of caution needs to be added. NEP also catalyses the breakdown of such adverse peptides as endothelin, a very potent vasoconstrictor. It might be that any beneficial effects of NEP inhibition will be counteracted by an increase in endothelin.

Conclusions

- Activation of the RAAS plays a significant role in the progression of chronic heart failure.

- ACE inhibitors improve symptoms and reduce mortality in chronic heart failure.

- Most evidence pertains to enalapril and captopril, but it is likely that this is a class effect.

- All patients with chronic heart failure should receive an ACE inhibitor unless specifically contraindicated.

- With few exceptions, ACE inhibitors can be started in the community, with appropriate monitoring.

- Larger doses are better than smaller doses.

- Spironolactone is indicated in patients with severe chronic heart failure and well-preserved renal function. K^+ should be regularly checked in such patients.

- New strategies, such as combined ACE inhibitor and angiotensin II receptor antagonist therapy and 'vasopeptidase inhibitors', continue to be developed.

References

1. Skeggs LT. Discovery of the two angiotensin peptides and the angiotensin-converting enzyme. *Hypertension* 1993; **21**: 259–260.

2. Laragh JH, Angers M, Kelly WG, Lieberman S. Hypotensive agents and pressor substances. The effect of epinephrine, norepinephrine, angiotensin II and others on the secretory rate of aldosterone in man. *J Am Med Assoc* 1960; **174**: 234–240.

3. Schorb W, Booz GW, Dostal DE et al. Angiotensin II is mitogenic in neonatal rat cardiac fibroblasts. *Circ Res* 1993; **72**: 1245–1254.

4. Hahn AWA, Schmidt R, Kern F et al. Endothelium-modulated proliferation of medial smooth muscle cells: influence of angiotensin II and converting enzyme inhibition. *Eur Heart J* 1995; **16 (Suppl C)**: 29–32.

5. Dubey RK, Jackson EK, Rupprecht HD, Sterzel RB. Factors controlling growth and matrix production in vascular muscle and glomerular mesangial cells. *Curr Op Neph Hypertens* 1997; **6**: 88 105.

6. Ito H, Adachi S, Tanaka M et al. Endothelin-1 is a paracrine/autocrine factor in the mechanism of angiotensin II-induced hypertrophy in cultured rat cardiomyocytes. *J Clin Invest* 1993; **92**: 398–403.

7. Wolf G, Mueller E, Stahl RA, Ziyadeh FN. Angiotensin II-induced hypertrophy of cultured murine proximal tubular cells is mediated by endogenous transforming growth factor-β. *J Clin Invest* 1993; **92**: 1366–1372.

8. Ferarri R, Ceconi C, Curello S, Visioli O. The neuroendocrine and sympathetic nervous system in congestive heart failure. *Eur Heart J* 1998; **19 (Suppl F)**: 45–51.

9. Teerlink JR. Neurohumoral mechanisms in heart failure: a central role for the renin–angiotensin system. *J Cardiovasc Pharm* 1996; **27 (Suppl 2)**: S1–S8.

10. Brilla CG, Rupp H, Funck R, Maisch B. The renin–angiotensin–aldosterone system and myocardial collagen matrix remodelling in

congestive heart failure. *Eur Heart J* 1995; **16** (**Suppl O**): 107–109.

11. The CONSENSUS Trial Study Group. Effects of enalapril on mortality in severe congestive heart failure. Results of the Cooperative North Scandinavian Enalapril Survival Study (CONSENSUS). *N Engl J Med* 1987; **316**: 747–752.

12. Swedburg K, Kjekshus J, Snapinn S for the CONSENSUS investigators. Long-term survival in severe heart failure in patients treated with enalapril. *Eur Heart J* 1999; **20**: 136–139.

13. The SOLVD Investigators. Effect of enalapril on survival in patients with reduced left ventricular ejection fractions and congestive heart failure. *N Engl J Med* 1991; **325**: 293–302.

14. The SOLVD Investigators. Effect of enalapril on mortality and the development of heart failure in asymptomatic patients with reduced left ventricular ejection fractions. *N Engl J Med* 1992; **327**: 685–691.

15. Cohn JN, Archibald DG, Ziesche S et al. Effect of vasodilator therapy on mortality in chronic congestive heart failure. *N Engl J Med* 1986; **314**: 1547–1552.

16. Cohn JN, Johnson G, Ziesche S et al. A comparison of enalapril with hydralazine-isosorbide dinitrate in the treatment of chronic congestive heart failure. *N Engl J Med* 1991; **325**: 303–310.

17. Garg R, Yusuf S. Overview of randomized trials of angiotensin-converting enzyme inhibitors on mortality and morbidity in patients with heart failure. Collaborative Group on ACE Inhibitor Trials. *J Am Med Assoc* 1995; **273**: 1450–1456.

18. Pfeffer MA, Braunwald E, Moye LA et al.

Effect of captopril on mortality and morbidity in patients with left ventricular dysfunction after myocardial infarction. Results of the Survival and Ventricular Enlargement trial (SAVE). *N Engl J Med* 1992; **327**: 669–677.

19. Kober L, Torp-Pedersson C, Carlsen JE et al. A clinical trial of the angiotensin-converting enzyme inhibitor trandolapril in patients with left ventricular dysfunction after myocardial infarction. *N Engl J Med* 1995; **333**: 1670–1676.

20. The Acute Infarction Ramipril Efficacy (AIRE) Study Investigators. Effect of ramipril on mortality and morbidity of survivors of acute myocardial infarction with clinical evidence of heart failure. *Lancet* 1993; **342**: 821–828.

21. Swedburg K, Held P, Rasmussen K et al. Effects of the early administration of enalapril on mortality in patients with acute myocardial infarction: results of the Cooperative New Scandinavian Enalapril Survival Study (CONSENSUS II). *N Engl J Med* 1992; **327**: 678–684.

22. ISIS-4 (Fourth International Study of Infarct Survival) Collaborative Group, ISIS-4. A randomized factorial trail assessing early oral captopril, oral mononitrate and intravenous magnesium in 58,050 patients with suspected acute myocardial infarction. *Lancet* 1995; **345**: 669–685.

23. Gruppo Italiano per Io studio della Sporavvivenza nell' Infarcto Miocardio (GISSI-3). Effects of lisinopril and transdermal glyceryl trinitrate singly and together on 6-week mortality and ventricular function after acute myocardial infarction. *Lancet* 1994; **343**: 1115–1122.

24. Ljungman S, Kjekshus J, Swedburg K, for the CONSENSUS Trial Group. Renal function

in severe congestive heart failure during treatment with enalapril (the Cooperative North Scandinavian Enalapril Survival Study [CONSENSUS] Trial). *Am J Cardiol* 1992; **70**: 479–487.

25. Packer M, Poole-Wilson PA, Armstrong PW et al. Comparative effects of low and high doses of the angiotensin-converting enzyme inhibitor, lisinopril, on morbidity and mortality in chronic heart failure. ATLAS Study Group. *Circulation* 1999; **100**: 2312–2318.

26. Biollaz J, Brunner HR, Gavras I et al. Antihypertensive treatment with MK 421: angiotensin II–renin relationships to evaluate efficacy of converting enzyme blockade. *J Cardiovasc Pharmacol* 1982; **4**: 966–972.

27. Rousseau MF, Konstam MA, Benedict CR et al. Progression of left ventricular dysfunction secondary to coronary artery disease, sustained neurohumoral activation and effects of ibopamine therapy during long term therapy with angiotensin-converting enzyme inhibitor. *Am J Cardiol* 1994; **73**: 488–493.

28. Lees KR. The dose response relationship with angiotensin-converting enzyme inhibitors: effects on blood pressure and biochemical parameters. *J Hypertens* 1992; **10** (**Suppl 5**): S3–S11.

29. Urata H, Healy B, Stewart RW et al. Angiotensin II-forming pathways in normal and failing human hearts. *Circ Res* 1990; **66**: 883–890.

30. Pitt B, Poole-Wilson P, Segal R et al., on behalf of the ELITE II investigators. Effect of losartan compared with captopril on mortality in patients with symptomatic heart failure: randomised trial—the Losartan Heart Failure Survival Study ELITE II. *Lancet* 2000; **355**: 1582–1587.

31. Cohn JN, Tognoni G, Glazer RD et al. Rationale and design of the Valsartan Heart Failure Trial: a large multinational trial to assess the effects of valsartan, an angiotensin-receptor blocker, on morbidity and mortality in chronic congestive heart failure. *J Card Fail* 1999; **5**: 155–160.

32. Swedberg K, Pfeffer M, Granger C et al. Candesartan in heart failure – assessment of reduction in mortality and morbidity (CHARM): rationale and design. CHARM-Programme Investigators. *J Card Fail* 1999; **5**: 276–282.

33. Azizi M, Guyenne T-T, Chatellier G et al. Additive effects of losartan and enalapril on blood pressure and plasma active renin. *Hypertension* 1997; **29**: 634–640.

34. Gainer JV, Morrow JD, Loveland A et al. Effect of bradykinin-receptor blockade on the response to angiotensin-converting enzyme inhibitor in normotensive and hypertensive subjects. *N Engl J Med* 1998; **339**: 1285–1292.

35. Hamroff G, Katz SD, Mancini D et al. Addition of angiotensin II receptor blockade to maximal angiotensin-converting enzyme inhibition improves exercise capacity in patients with severe congestive heart failure. *Circulation* 1999; **99**: 990–992.

36. Pitt B, Zannad F, Remme WJ et al. The effect of spironolactone on morbidity and mortality in patients with severe heart failure. *N Engl J Med* 1999; **341**: 709–717.

37. Trippodo NC, Fox M, Monticello TM et al. Vasopeptidase inhibition with omapatrilat improves cardiac geometry in cardiomyopathic hamsters more than does ACE inhibition with captopril. *J Cardiovasc Pharmacol* 1999; **34**: 782–790.

38. Rouleau JL, Pfeffer MA, Stewart DJ et al. Comparison of vasopeptidase inhibitor, omapatrilat and lisinopril on exercise tolerance and morbidity in patients with heart failure: IMPRESS randomised trial. *Lancet* 2000; **356**: 615–620.

Inhibitors of the sympathetic nervous system

Samuel J McClure

8

Increased activity of the sympathetic nervous system (SNS) is an essential physiological reaction to environmental changes: even postural change would not be possible without a rapid SNS response. Over the past three decades it has become clear that a sustained and inappropriate SNS activation accompanies[1-4] and, more importantly, contributes to[5,6] the progression of chronic heart failure.

Modulation of SNS activity is now being extensively investigated in heart failure, and β-adrenoceptor antagonism has been convincingly shown to improve prognosis in stable chronic heart failure. The use of other SNS inhibitors is at an earlier stage of evaluation.

Sympathetic activation in chronic heart failure

That worsening severity of heart failure is associated with increasing urinary noradrenaline (norepinephrine) excretion has been recognized for many years.[1] Subsequently, elevated plasma noradrenaline concentration was reported.[2] These findings were initially thought to be simply a marker of heart failure. A seminal work by Cohn et al demonstrated a striking correlation between high plasma noradrenaline concentration and worse prognosis in chronic heart failure patients.[7]

Technical developments have enabled direct methods to be used for SNS assessment such as microneurography[8] (direct intraneural recordings of, for example, peroneal sympathetic nerve traffic). Microneurography has confirmed that SNS activity correlates with cardiac index, stroke volume index, and systemic and pulmonary vascular resistances, although it is not related to ejection fraction.[9] Modern indirect methods of SNS assessment such as measurement of heart rate variability[10] and plasma 'spillover' of noradrenaline[11] collectively confirm that SNS activity is progressively increased, and parasympathetic activity blunted,[12,13] as left ventricular dysfunction develops into clinical chronic heart failure and the syndrome increases in severity. Although SNS activity is related to severity of heart failure, an irrefutable demonstration that increased SNS output directly causes or contributes to the decline in cardiac performance and disease progression remains elusive.

The 'neurohormonal hypothesis' of heart failure attributes clinical manifestations and progression of chronic heart failure to abnormal modulation of neurohormonal systems.[14] Increased plasma concentrations of renin, angiotensin, endothelins and catecholamines do not just accompany the condition, but cause and perpetuate it. This understanding has

developed after the success of angiotensin converting enzyme (ACE) inhibitors.[15–17] ACE inhibitors have beneficial effects over and above those achieved by drugs that simply vasodilate (the main haemodynamic effect of ACE inhibitors.[1,18] The hypothesis has been further bolstered by the results of several trials of β-blockers (see below).

Recently, the RALES Trial using spironolactone at a dose chosen to block aldosterone receptors has also proven significant mortality benefits in CHF,[19] again adding weight to the neurohormonal hypothesis.

Neurohormonal hypothesis

Increased activity of neurohormonal systems such as the renin–angiotensin–aldosterone system (RAAS) and the SNS is an appropriate and essential response to preserve circulatory homeostasis in the short term after an insult that reduces cardiac output. However, unlike other clinical situations such as hypovolaemia, where cardiac output may be reduced temporarily, ventricular damage is not normally reversible and stimulation of systems such as the RAAS and SNS persists. The counterregulatory vasodilator, natriuretic and diuretic responses (such as increased plasma concentrations of natriuretic peptides and perhaps adrenomedullin) do not adequately oppose this activity during permanent ventricular dysfunction.

Subsequent chronic imbalance of neurohormonal systems occurs, cardiac workload increases (owing to increased heart rate, peripheral vasoconstriction and fluid retention), and results in a progressive decline in circulatory performance and the clinical features of chronic heart failure. The effects of oxidative stress (known to increase in chronic heart failure), increased apoptosis and elevated concentrations of cytokines may also contribute to disease progression. Successful drugs like the ACE inhibitors alter the unbalanced neurohormonal melieu from vasoconstricted, inotropic and fluid retaining to a more beneficial vasodilated, less inotropic and more diuretic state. SNS inhibitors might further improve this balance.

Sympathomimetic agents

It was long believed that cardiac stimulation by inotropes would support circulatory function when chronically impaired ventricular performance was present. Catecholamines are depleted in the failing heart, which suggests that exogenous catecholamines might be beneficial. Beta-adrenoceptor density is decreased (and thus endogenous catecholamine responsiveness reduced) in chronic heart failure, so a logical step would be the use of therapeutic agents to enhance endogenous adrenergic activity.

However, clinical trials have shown that several sympathomimetic positive inotropic agents such as dobutamine (β_1-agonist),[20]

levodopa (dopamine agonist),[21] xamoterol (partial β_1-agonist)[22] and phosphodiesterase inhibitors (acting via SNS second messenger systems)[23–26] increase the mortality rate in chronic heart failure. Whilst such drugs could often improve symptoms and measures of cardiac function in the short term,[27] they contributed to progressive decline in the long term.[20,28] A summary of the drugs tried and their actions is provided in *Table 8.1*.

Inotropic support for the failing heart is not the way forward. It might be that the attenuated ability of myocardium to respond to continuously high levels of endogenous or exogenous catecholamines is a natural counterregulatory attempt to withdraw from unhelpful influences. Agents that further withdraw SNS influences from the circulation might be beneficial.

Reducing sympathetic nervous system activity in chronic heart failure

Inhibition of sympathetic traffic to the heart and peripheral vasculature may be accomplished by various means (see *Figure 8.1*):

1. Blocking post-synaptic α and β receptors.
2. Activating central nervous system areas to inhibit SNS outflow.
3. Ganglion-blocking drugs. These interrupt transmission in the sympathetic ganglia by

Table 8.1
Drugs enhancing natural adrenergic activity which result in an increased mortality in chronic heart failure

Drug	Reference	Mode of action	Potency
Xamoterol	22	β-Receptor agonist	+ +
Dobutamine	20	Dopamine, α, β agonist	+ + +
Ibopamine	86	Dopamine, α, β agonist	+
Amrinone	23	Phosphodiesterase inhibitor	+ + +
Enoximone	87	Phosphodiesterase inhibitor	+ + +
Milrinone	24	Phosphodiesterase inhibitor	+ + +
Piroximone	25	Phosphodiesterase inhibitor	+ +
Fenoximone	26	Phosphodiesterase inhibitor	+ +
Levodopa	29	Dopamine agonist	+ +
Vesnarinone	30	Phosphodiesterase inhibitor	+ +
Flosequinan	88	Attenuates inositol triphosphate	+

blockade of nicotinic cholinergic receptors (hexamethonium, pentapyrrolidinium). Unfortunately, drugs in this class block almost all autonomic outflow at both sympathetic and parasympathetic ganglia, and thus produce such a wide range of side-effects as to make routine use impossible. Short reports indicated a worsening in heart failure with pentapyrrolidinium.[29]

4. Depletion of inactivation of noradrenaline stores in the peripheral postganglionic sympathetic neurones using, for example, guanethidine or reserpine. These drugs also worsened heart failure in small studies.[30]

5. Inhibition of tyrosine hydroxylase to reduce production of catecholamines: one small study of the use of metyrosine for this purpose exists.[31] Whilst a decrease in plasma noradrenaline concentration was observed, no haemodynamic effect was found and the study was taken by the authors to show no influence in chronic heart failure.

Only drugs in the first two classes are available for routine use. This chapter concentrates on the experience so far with β-receptor antagonists and the use of central SNS inhibitors in the treatment of chronic heart failure.

Alpha-blockers in heart failure

When the haemodynamic hypothesis of heart failure dominated treatment strategies, vasodilatation to reduce cardiac preload and afterload was the therapeutic goal. Various approaches to vasodilatation were pursued,

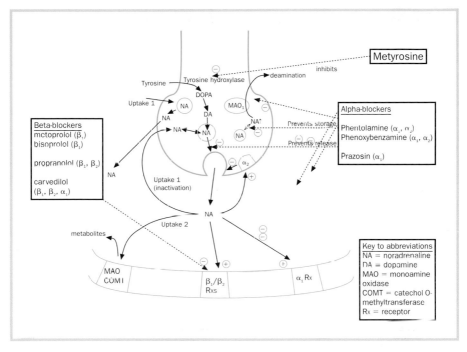

Figure 8.1
Diagram of a sympathetic nerve terminal with sites of action of some drugs

including α-adrenergic receptor antagonism, which produces sustained vasodilatation by blocking the vasoconstriction caused by SNS activity.

Oral administration of phentolamine[32] and phenoxybenzamine[33] (non-selective α-blockers, with action on both pre- and post-synaptic α-receptors) produced acute haemodynamic improvement in early observational reports. However, phentolamine causes reflex stimulation of the sympathetic neurones, resulting in greater overall transmitter release and heightened stimulation of β-receptors, consequently accelerating heart rate. Phenoxybenzamine also produces tachycardia, by reducing presynaptic reuptake of noradrenaline (for site of action of these drugs, see *Figure 8.1*).

The selective α₁-blockers, prazosin[34] and trimazosin,[35] give short-term haemodynamic benefits, tolerance to the acute haemodynamic effects develops, and there is no clinical benefit after longer-term usage.[36] In particular, prazosin was found to produce no sustained haemodynamic or mortality benefit in chronic heart failure,[37,38] and actually increased the circulating concentration of noradrenaline and caused salt and water retention.[39,40] Doxazosin has a more prolonged duration of action than earlier members of the class. Recently, the ALLHAT (Antihypertensive and Lipid-lowering Treatment to Prevent Heart Attack Trial) study[41] had its doxazosin-treatment arm discontinued, owing to a significant increase in the numbers of patients developing congestive heart failure. This clearly calls the use of α-blockers in chronic heart failure into further question; it is unlikely that further such trials will be attempted.

Beta-blockers in heart failure

The conventional view of β-blockers is that they depress cardiac performance via negative inotropy and negative chronotropy, and thus worsen chronic heart failure. Swedish work more than 20 years ago contradicted this view,[42] but was not widely accepted. A number of small-scale clinical trials at this time were inconclusive and certainly did not encourage further development; inotrope and vasodilator development was in vogue, and progress appeared to lie in these directions. Beta-blockers were thus virtually abandoned as chronic heart failure therapy until the 1990s.

The enormous success of ACE inhibitors in large-scale clinical trials helped evolve the neurohormonal hypothesis of chronic heart failure. For the first time, the emphasis in these trials was not necessarily to detect an improvement in patient symptoms, at least in the short term, but was rather to detect an improvement in mortality which might suggest a delay in disease progression. This finally led to a number of clinical trials of β-blocking agents.

The first Swedish trials were observational,[42] whilst during the 1980s, surrogate outcome variables were employed such as exercise tolerance and change in ejection fraction, rather than mortality. Results using different agents seemed variable, which did little to bolster the case for β-blockade. Experience with ACE inhibitor trials showed that larger-scale trials were required, and after the worsening mortality seen in the inotrope trials, the consensus developed that the primary end-point of trials should be an influence on mortality rates. Huge numbers of patients are required for such studies, so that enough end-points occur to reveal genuine differences between groups.

Patients enrolled in the β-blocker studies were usually already treated with the conventional heart failure therapy, usually comprising ACE inhibitors and diuretics. In some trials, there was also a significant frequency of treatment with digoxin. For a summary of the large β-blocker trials, see *Table 8.2.*

Table 8.2
Summary of results from the large β-blocker trials

	MDC (no IHD patients)[43]		CIBIS-I[89]		US carvedilol trials[46-49]		A-NZ carvedilol trials[56]		CIBIS-II[51]		MERIT-HF[57]	
	Placebo	Metoprolol	Placebo	Metoprolol	Placebo	Carvedilol	Placebo	Carvedilol	Placebo	Bisoprolol	Placebo	Metoprolol
n	189	194	321	320	398	696	208	207	1320	1327	2001	1990
Mean age (years)	49	49	59	60	58	58	67	67	61	61	64	64
Male (%)	75	70	83	83	76	77	85	76	80	51	78	77
NYHA I (%)	—	—	—	—	—	—	30	30	—	—	—	—
NYHA II (%)	47	42	0	0	52	54	49	59	—	—	41	41
NYHA III (%)	47	51	95	95	44	44	21	11	83	83	55	56
NYHA IV (%)	4	4	5	5	3	3	—	—	17	17	4	3
LVEF (%)	22	22	26	25	22	23	29	28	28	28	28	28
IHD (%)	0	0	53	56	47	47	89	88	50	50	66	65
Hypertension (%)	—	—	—	—	—	—	—	—	—	—	44	44
AF (%)	—	—	14	12.5	—	—	—	—	20	20	17	16
Angina (%)	0	0	35	38	—	—	25	24	—	—	—	—
ACE inhibitor (%)	82	78	91	89	95	95	85	86	96	96	90	89
Mean follow-up (months)	16 (approximately)		23		6.5 (median)		19		16		12	
Hospitalization (n)	83	51	90	61	19.6%	14.1%	120	99	39	33	—	—
Transplantation (n)	12	2	6	3	—	—	—	—	—	—	—	—
Mortality (%)	11	12	21	17	7.8	3.2	12.5	9.7	17.3	11.8	11.0	7.2
Absolute risk reduction	—		—		4.6		—		5.5		3.8	
Relative risk reduction (%)	—		—		65		—		34		34	
p Value	Not significant		Not significant		<0.001		Not significant		<0.0001		0.00009	

The Metoprolol in Dilated Cardiomyopathy (MDC) study[43] randomized 383 patients on standard treatment to either metoprolol or placebo. Follow-up was for 12–18 months. There was no significant effect on total mortality, but there was an effect that almost reached statistical significance on the combined end-point of mortality or progression to cardiac transplantation. There was a non-significant excess of deaths seen in the metoprolol-treated group.

The Cardiac Insufficiency Bisoprolol Study (CIBIS-I)[44] randomized 641 patients with heart failure (NYHA II-IV) of various aetiologies to bisoprolol or placebo for a mean follow-up period of 1.9 years. Again, there was no significant difference between groups in mortality, but fewer bisoprolol-treated patients required hospitalization, and more showed improvement in function class. Subgroup analysis suggested that benefit from β-blockade therapy was greater for those with non-ischaemic cardiomyopathy, which at the time of publication appeared to add support to the view that idiopathic cardiomyopathy patients had more to gain from β-blocker therapy.

The key publication of the US carvedilol trials persuaded large sections of the cardiology community of the value of β-blockade in heart failure.[45] The publication was the amalgamated results from four smaller studies,[46–49] with a total of 1094 patients enrolled for 6.5 months. Details of the studies and their planned primary end-points are shown in *Table 8.3*. It showed a 65%

Table 8.3
Details of the US carvedilol study components

	References	Number of patients	Proportion of patients treated with carvedilol : placebo	Primary end-point
Mild CHF	*46*	*366*	*2 : 1*	*Progession of CHF*
MOCHA	*48*	*345*	*3 : 1*	*Exercise tolerance*
PRECISE	*47*	*278*	*1 : 1*	*Exercise tolerance*
Severe CHF	*49*	*105*	*2 : 1*	*Quality of life*

CHF, chronic heart failure.

reduction in mortality (95% confidence intervals of 39–80%) with carvedilol. The improved prognosis occurred regardless of heart failure aetiology. A common data and safety monitoring board monitored the collective mortality in the four separate trials (with separate efficacy end-points) and the decision was taken to terminate the trials early, owing to the marked reduction in mortality.

In addition to effects on mortality, carvedilol reduced the proportion of patients requiring hospitalization for a cardiovascular cause (risk reduction 27% with 95% confidence intervals of 3–45%). The proportions admitted for any cause and for worsening chronic heart failure were also significantly reduced. Tolerability of carvedilol seems broadly similar to that of other β-blockers in chronic heart failure, although dizziness is perhaps more common.

The study was, however, an amalgam of four smaller studies, none of which had been powered to look at mortality. Follow-up was short, and the number of clinical events was very small.

The ANZ (carvedilol) trial enrolled 415 patients with mild chronic heart failure randomized to placebo or carvedilol.[50] There was a non-significant reduction in mortality at 18 months: lack of significance has been attributed to the relatively good prognosis for patients with mild chronic heart failure.

The landmark CIBIS-II (bisoprolol) study was the first randomized, double-blind, placebo-controlled trial of a β-blocker in heart failure with sufficient power to address all-cause mortality as a primary end-point.[51] The large number of patients and the large number of deaths in the study (384 in CIBIS-II compared with 54 in the US carvedilol studies) make the data much more robust than the carvedilol studies. CIBIS-II was the first study to provide conclusive evidence in favour of β-blockers, or at least bisoprolol, in heart failure. A total of 2647 ambulatory, mostly male, patients said to have NYHA grade III or IV heart failure of ischaemic or non-ischaemic aetiology and left ventricular ejection fraction of ≤35% were recruited. The study was halted early, with average follow-up of 1.4 years, owing to a highly significant mortality reduction in favour of bisoprolol. A fall of 34% in all-cause mortality ($p < 0.0001$) was seen, and of particular note was the 45% reduction in sudden death.

Bisoprolol also achieved a significant effect on cardiovascular morbidity, with fewer bisoprolol-treated patients (33%) requiring a hospital admission as compared with placebo (39%). Hospital admission for worsening heart failure was also reduced to 12% from 18% in the placebo group. Tolerability of the medication was the same (15% discontinued) in both the placebo and the treatment groups.

MERIT-HF (metoprolol CR/XL) is the largest trial so far published of β blockers in heart failure, and has been particularly encouraging as its results are highly consistent with those of CIBIS-II and with meta-analyses of previous β-blocker trials. The 3991 patients included were in NYHA functional class II-IV, had left ventricular ejection fractions of <40% and were all on standard heart failure therapy. Use of a long-acting form of metoprolol produced a 34% reduction in mortality after a mean follow-up time of 1 year. Like CIBIS-II, the large study size and large number of events (362 deaths) would suggest that the data are robust. An independent safety committee recommended early completion of the study, owing to the magnitude of benefit seen in the treated group. Both suddent deaths and deaths due to heart failure were reduced. Tolerability of the drug was very similar to that of placebo (15.3% of the placebo group discontinued because of side-effects, compared to 13.9% of the metoprolol group).

The COPERNICUS study in patients with severe (NYHA class IIIb/iv) heart failure has recently shown a 35% reduction in mortality with carvedilol.

Bucindolol is another β-blocker with vasodilating properties that has been evaluated in heart failure patients.[52–54] Preliminary results from the BEST (Beta-Blocker Evaluation of Survival Trial) study suggest no statistically significant benefit of treatment on all-cause mortality.[55] This was an unexpected result, with only a non-significant trend toward benefit in patients with moderate to severe heart failure: mortality was reduced by 10% on bucindolol as compared with placebo ($p = 0.109$). This magnitude of benefit is considerably less than that seen in CIBIS-II and MERIT-HF. A higher proportion of patients had severe heart failure (recruitment was open to patients with NYHA class III-IV) in BEST than in CIBIS II or MERIT-HF, and the ethnicity of the patients was different (whilst CIBIS II and MERIT-HF had predominantly Caucasian subjects, BEST had a 23% African-American complement).[56] Subgroup analysis showed that, in patients with NYHA III heart failure or left ventricular ejection fraction of >20%, improved survival occurred, but there was no benefit in those with left ventricular ejection fraction of <20% or in NYHA IV. Of particular note was a non-statistically significant excess mortality in the African-American subgroup. Commentators have suggested that future studies should pay more attention to the ethnicity of the study population, as there may in fact be differences between racial groups in their response to therapy.

Bucindolol cannot therefore be recommended as a treatment option in chronic heart failure. This opens the questions as to whether the benefits of β-blockers in chronic heart failure are a 'class effect', whether there are specific properties of some β-blockers that are more desirable, or whether bucindolol has some peculiar adverse property. Bucindolol has intrinsic sympathomimetic activity, and comparison might be made with xamoterol, a β-blocker with marked sympathomimetic properties.[22]

Effects of β-blockers on morbidity and quality of life

Although β-blockers prolong life, the effect on quality of life and morbidity is, of course, also important. Some positive inotropes reduce survival in chronic heart failure, but improve quality of life; whilst patients might live longer on β-blockers, would there be a reduction in quality of life so as to make this new therapy unacceptable?

There is, in fact, a consistent improvement in quality of life in the large β-blocker studies. Variables used to assess quality of life have been frequency of hospitalizations, NYHA class, symptom scores or global assessment by the patient and their physician. The reduction in hospitalization frequency is striking in both CIBIS-II and MERIT-HF,[57] and this variable is not usually susceptible to observer bias.

Choice of β-blocker

Whether all β-blockers have the same effect or whether there is a 'best β-blocker' remains undecided. Bisoprolol, metoprolol and carvedilol are the drugs with most evidence to support their use.

Mechanism of action

Which action of β-blockers is responsible for slowing chronic heart failure progression? Possible mechanisms include:

1. Blockade of the direct toxic effects of catecholamines,[58,59] particularly with the less selective β-blockers;
2. Reduction of systemic vascular resistance (SVR); in the short term, most β-blockers actually increase SVR, but the SVR is decreased after long-term administration,[60] presumably owing to improved myocardial performance or a decrease in sympathetic drive;
3. Antiarrhythmic action;[61]
4. Reduced renin secretion;[62]
5. Prolonged diastolic filling permitting increased effective myocardial blood flow;
6. Reduced myocardial ischaemia;
7. Slowing of heart rate, resulting in lower myocardial energy expenditure.

The last mechanism of action is particularly attractive, as perhaps simply 'resting the weary heart' is all that is required. Increased heart rate itself is an independent risk factor for death in chronic heart failure (and, indeed, in a variety of cardiovascular conditions).[63] The relative risk of all-cause mortality increases with increasing heart rate; this effect is restricted to cardiovascular causes of mortality and does not apply, for example, to cancer mortality.[64] Positively inotropic medication to treat chronic heart failure produced increases in heart rate. Whether increased heart rate is simply an indicator of poorly treated chronic heart failure, or indicates increased risk, has not yet been clearly determined.

Initiating β-blocker treatment in chronic heart failure

Initiation of treatment with β-blockers in heart failure must be cautious.[65] Patients should have stable, compensated heart failure; β-blockers are not appropriate for those with overt pulmonary or peripheral oedema.

The great majority of patients enrolled in the large-scale clinical trials have had NYHA II or NYHA III heart failure. Some data now exist in NYHA IV patients, and some smaller trials[66] and meta-analyses have suggested benefit in this group. These conclusions are supported by the findings of the COPERNICUS trial. Less well patients are more likely to develop adverse events during initiation and dose titration,[66] but these less well patients may have most to gain. Until further data are available, NYHA class II and III patients should all be treated with β-blockers unless there are contraindications. There are no guidelines to help identify those patients most likely to have a favourable response to therapy. A resting tachycardia or

some other indicator of increased SNS activity might predict improvement on β-blockade but there is as yet no evidence to support this.

The initial dose should be low (far less than the dose used conventionally in hypertension or angina) and dose increases should be carried out under careful supervision, usually at 2-weekly intervals. By slow up-titration, the supportive role of SNS activity for the circulation is only slowly withdrawn. Carvedilol should be started at 3.125 mg twice a day, and bisoprolol at 1.25 mg once a day.

The only two β-blockers licensed for use in chronic heart failure in the UK are carvedilol and bisoprolol, both of which are now commercially available in the doses employed in the chronic heart failure studies. Metoprolol is not licensed for chronic heart failure, and indeed the long-acting preparation used in MERIT-HF is not yet available in the UK. Whether this long-acting form is required for the beneficial effect seen is certainly open to debate.[67]

Even with careful initiation there may be short-term decompensation requiring increases in the dose of diuretics. In the case of vasodilating β-blockers, symptoms of hypotension may require a decreased diuretic dose.

Central inhibition of sympathetic nervous system activity

More effective than simply blocking the end-organ effects of an overactive SNS might be inhibiting sympathetic output from its brain stem source. In this way, as well as reducing noradrenaline output, the release of other vasoconstrictor substances from nerve terminals might be reduced.

Centrally mediated modulation of the SNS has been available for many years in the form of clonidine, α-methyldopa, guanabenz and guanfacine. These medications have never been subjected to significant placebo-controlled trials, despite encouraging preliminary data in small studies.[68-70]

Treatment of hypertension with centrally acting drugs originated with the use of α-methyldopa in the 1960s. This pro-drug was quickly recognized as having its predominant effect within the central nervous system. Clonidine became the main drug of this class to be used in hypertension, as it is better tolerated. However, clonidine has side-effects: sedation (due to the central α_2 effect), dry mouth, fatigue and impotence (due to the peripheral α_2 effect) are common.

There were also two important theoretical concerns about the use of clonidine in chronic heart failure:

1. Anxiety about negative inotropism (due to withdrawal of the positive inotropic effect of catecholamines) in chronic heart failure, the same concern that for so long prevented β-blocker use in chronic heart failure. The fact that clonidine reduces preload[71] was taken as confirming negative inotropy. With the benefit of hindsight, this property may be a valuable asset for a chronic heart failure drug.

2. There was also concern about rebound effects (tachycardia and increase in blood pressure) when clonidine was withdrawn, and anecdotal evidence supported these concerns in heart failure.[72]

A number of small-scale studies of clonidine in chronic heart failure were conducted at a time when other vasodilators were becoming established. Despite some encouraging early results, there was no impetus to conduct larger scale trials. The 'haemodynamic hypothesis' of heart failure seemed to explain why vasodilator medication improved the condition. For a summary of studies of the classical central SNS inhibitors, see *Table 8.4*.

Mechanism of central action

The blood pressure-lowering actions of clonidine were thought to be mediated via central α_2 receptor agonism, resulting in reduced pre- and post-ganglionic discharge in the sympathetic nerves to heart and blood vessels, and facilitation of the vagal

Table 8.4
Summary of chronic heart failure studies using classical centrally acting antiadrenergic drugs

Drug	Author	Patients	HR	MAP	PCWP	PAP	SVR	PVR	CO/EF	NA	A	PRA	Other
Methyldopa	Kirlin et al. 1986[90]	14 NYHA II-III	↓	↓	ND	ND	↔	ND	↔	↓	↔	↑	No ↑ ET No ↓ NYHA
Guanabenz	Olivari et al. 1986[91]	10 NYHA III-IV	↓	↓	↓	↓	↔	↓	↔	↓	ND	↔	
Clonidine	Giles et al. 1985[92]	12	↓	↓	↓	↓	↓	↓	↑	↓	ND	ND	↑ SV
Guanabenz	Giles et al. 1985[92]	8	↓	ND	↓	ND	ND	ND	↔	↓	ND	ND	↓ RAP
Clonidine (chronic)	Giles et al. 1985[92]	10	↓	ND	ND	ND	ND	ND	↑	↓	ND	ND	↓ RAP, ↑ exercise tolerance
Clonidine	Good et al. 1988[93]	24 NYHA III-IV	↓	↓	↓	↓	↔	↓	↔	↓	ND	ND	
Clonidine	Hermiller et al. 1983[71]	14 NYHA III-IV	↓	↓	↓	↓	↓ (one dose)	↓	↑	ND	ND	ND	↓ RAP
Clonidine	Magorien et al. 1985[94]	10 NYHA III-IV	↓	↓	↓	↓	↓ NS	ND	↔	ND	ND	ND	
Clonidine (single dose)	Manolis et al. 1995[68]	20 NYHA III-IV	↓	↓	↓	ND	↓ NS	ND	↔	↓	↔	↓ NS	↓ NS
Clonidine (1-week therapy)	Manolis et al. 1995 (same patients as last study)[68]	7 NYHA III-IV	↔	↔	↓	ND	↔	ND	↓ NS	↓	↔	↓ NS	↓ NS
Clonidine + captopril (one dose)	Manolis et al. 1997[70]	9 NYHA III-IV	↓	↓	↓	↓	↓	↓	CI ↔	↓	↓ NS	↑	

Table 8.4
Continued

Drug	Author	Patients	HR	MAP	PCWP	PAP	SVR	PVR	CO/EF	NA	A	PRA	Other
Clonidine (single i.v. dose)	Lang et al. 1997[95]	20 NYHA III	→	→	→	→	↔	ND	↔	→	ND	ND	↓ pulmonary artery lactate during exercise ↓ Vo_2 max
Clonidine (single i.v. dose)	Azevedo et al. 1999[83]	9 NYHA II-III	→	→	NC	→	ND	NC	↔	→	ND	ND	

HR   = heart rate
MAP   = mean arterial pressure
PCWP   = pulmonary capillary wedge pressure
PAP   = pulmonary arterial pressure
SVR   = systemic vascular resistance
PVR   = pulmonary vascular resistance
CO/EF = cardiac output/ejection fraction
NA   = noradrenaline
A   = adrenaline
ET   = exercise tolerance
PRA   = plasma renin activity
RAP   = right atrial pressure
SV   = stroke volume
NYHA   = New York Heart Association functional class (cf heart failure)
SBP   = systolic blood pressure
ND   = not done
NS   = not significant

baroreceptor reflex. A new class of receptors has been recognized, both centrally and in peripheral SNS-related tissues, distinct from classic α-adrenergic receptors, and specific for imidazoline-like compounds.[73,74] The blood pressure-reducing effect of centrally acting antihypertensives correlates with their affinity to the 'imidazoline recognition sites' rather than with their affinity to α_2 receptors.

The imidazoline receptors have been subdivided into imidazoline receptor type 1 (I_1) and type 2 (I_2) subtypes. I_1 receptors have a restricted distribution within the central nervous system (mainly the rostral ventrolateral medulla; RVLM) and some related tissue (notably, the adrenal medulla).[75] The RVLM is an area crucially involved in the baroreceptor reflex, and animal studies show that this is the point at which most centrally acting antiadrenergics exert their hypotensive influence.

Already marketed for treatment of hypertension for several years, moxonidine is believed to be a relatively specific agonist at I_1 receptors (with very little action on α_2 receptors) with effects to reduce sympathetic outflow from the brain stem through action at the RVLM (*Figure 8.2*).[76] The specificity of moxonidine for I_1 receptors with minimal effect on α_2 receptors means that the drug has few clonidine-like side-effects (*Figure 8.3*). Moxonidine is well tolerated in hypertension, with a potency comparable to that of all the major classes of antihypertensive in current

clinical usage.[77] A summary of published data from moxonidine studies in chronic heart failure is in *Table 8.5*.

Centrally acting sympathetic nervous system inhibitors in chronic heart failure

Centrally acting antiadrenergic agents offer the opportunity of reducing systemic vascular resistance to offset the potential negative inotropism of withdrawing cardiac adrenergic drive. This reduced drive might be detectable by, for example, a lowered plasma noradrenaline concentration.

An attractive feature of centrally acting antiadrenergic drugs is that circulatory reflexes are left largely intact despite the depression of peripheral sympathetic activity. Both clonidine and moxonidine cause a fall in blood pressure, owing to a reduction in peripheral vascular resistance due in turn to inhibition of central adrenergic tone. Both drugs act to reset the sensitivity of the baroreceptor reflex (baroreceptor sensitivity is reduced in chronic heart failure). This action may explain the improvement in heart rate variability (shown to be an important predictive factor for mortality in chronic heart failure) seen with both moxonidine and clonidine.[78] Haemodynamic studies confirm clonidine as a potential adjunctive therapy to ACE inhibitors,[70,79] and it is safe in acute dosing.[80,81]

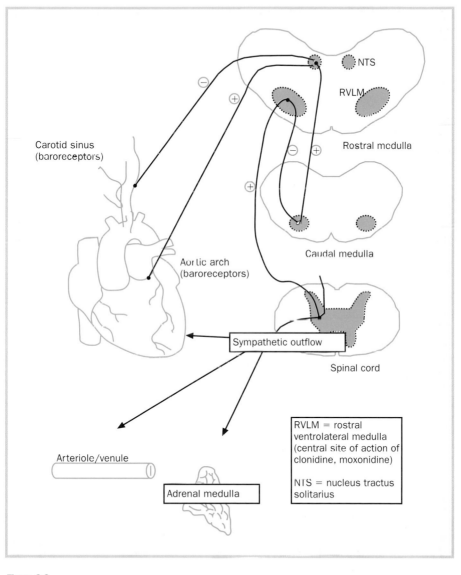

Figure 8.2
The baroreceptor reflex and its role in haemodynamic homeostasis

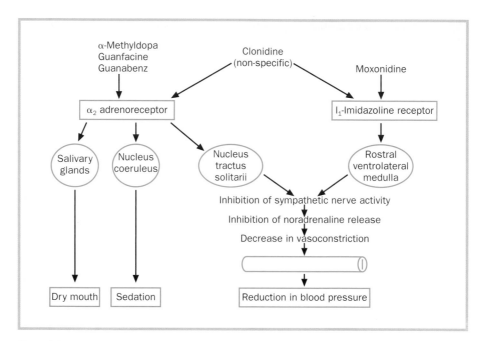

Figure 8.3
Sites and modes of action of central SNS inhibitors

A decrease in cardiac and peripheral (muscle) sympathetic activity in healthy human volunteers, assessed by microneurography, has been demonstrated with orally administered moxonidine.[82] Clonidine is effective in reducing sympathetic activity, and particularly cardiac sympathetic activity, in human heart failure.[83] The effect of clonidine on cardiac sympathetic activity is much greater than that seen with β-blockers. Moxonidine causes a marked reduction in the plasma concentration of noradrenaline in idiopathic dilated cardiomyopathy,[80] and a pilot study using sustained-release moxonidine in chronic heart failure (MOXSE) has also confirmed reduced noradrenaline levels.[84] Statistically significant reductions in plasma concentrations of angiotensin II have also been observed in heart failure patients during treatment with moxonidine.

Abrupt withdrawal of clonidine resulting in rebound activation of the SNS is a significant clinical problem. The severe tachycardia, rhythmic upswings of blood

Table 8.5
Summary of studies so far published/presented of moxonidine in chronic heart failure

Drug	Author	Patients	HR	MAP	PCWP	PAP	SVR	PVR	CO/EF	NE	E	PRA	Other
Moxonidine (single dose)	Mitrovic et al. 1996[80]	10 NYHA II-III (All IDC)	↓	↓	ND	↓↑	↓ NS	ND	↓	↓	↓ NS	↓ NS	↓ Angiotensin II No change in exercise capacity
Moxonidine	Swedberg et al. 1997[96]	69 NYHA II-III, 3 different doses	↓ (high dose only)	(SBP) ↓ NS	ND	ND	ND	ND	ND	↓	ND	ND	
Moxonidine (single dose)	Dickstein et al. 1997[97]	20 NYHA III	ND	↓	↓	ND	↓	↓	ND	↓	ND	ND	
Moxonidine (single dose)	Dickstein et al. 1999[91]	20 NYHA III	↓	↓	↓	↓	↓	↓	ND	↓	ND	ND	

HR   = heart rate
MAP   = mean arterial pressure
PCWP   = pulmonary capillary wedge pressure
PAP   = pulmonary arterial pressure
SVR   = systemic vascular resistance
PVR   = pulmonary vascular resistance
CO/EF = cardiac output/ejection fraction
NA   = noradrenaline
A   = adrenaline
ET   = exercise tolerance
PRA   = plasma renin activity
RAP   = right atrial pressure
SV   = stroke volume
NYHA   = New York Heart Association functional class (of heart failure)
SBP   = systolic blood pressure
ND   = not done
NS   = not significant

pressure and rise in plasma noradrenaline level in animal models of clonidine withdrawal is reflected by clinical experience in humans, particularly in chronic heart failure.[72] No comparable effects after withdrawal of moxonidine have been noted either in animal models or in human experiments. The usual side-effects of clonidine, i.e. sedation, dry mouth and impotence, are much less marked during treatment with moxonidine. The MOXSE pilot study in chronic heart failure has confirmed the good tolerability of moxonidine.[84]

However, large-scale trials, powered adequately to show an influence on mortality, are required before a new chronic heart failure therapy can be introduced. Whether centrally acting antiadrenergics are as effective as β-blockers in improving prognosis, or whether they could safely be used in addition to β-blockers in patients already treated with ACE inhibitors, remains to be established.

The first large-scale trial of moxonidine, the MOXCON (Sustained Release Moxonidine for Congestive Heart Failure) study has been terminated early, owing to increased mortality rates in the treatment group.[85] The Data and Safety Monitoring Board discontinued the study when only 2000 of the planned 4540 patients had been enrolled, owing to the deaths of 53 patients in the treatment group compared to 29 in the placebo group, most deaths being sudden. There was also a greater number of

hospitalizations for worsening heart failure, acute myocardial infarction and other adverse events. It is not yet clear why these effects were seen, but it was noted during the study that the plasma noradrenaline concentration fell to subphysiological levels in some patients; the drug had a greater-than-expected effect on noradrenaline levels.

The full MOXCON data are not yet published, but the use of centrally acting agents, particularly sustained-release moxonidine, is not currently recommended in chronic heart failure. Some commentators have argued that this result has cast some doubt on the hypothesis that SNS activation is causative in chronic heart failure, others that the dose of moxonidine used in the trial was equivalent to starting treatment with a high dose of a β-blocker, rather than a gradual titration from a low starting dose. Further large studies will be required to clarify the situation.

Other approaches

Many of the other drugs used in the treatment of heart failure modulate the SNS. Diuretics, for example, activate the SNS. Inhibition of the RAS decreases the potentiation of the SNS by angiotensin II and aldosterone. Amiodarone also has antiadrenergic properties.

Other therapeutic approaches may have some impact on the SNS. Exercise training partially reverses sympathetic : parasympathetic imbalance.[98] Treatment might be aimed at excessively active chemoreceptors, and potentially at the under-active baroreceptors in heart failure. Digoxin, for example, exerts an antiadrenergic effect[99] in parallel with a return of the baroreflex sensitivity towards normal.[100]

Conclusions

Activation of the SNS is an important component of the chronic heart failure syndrome, and seems to be responsible in part for the progression of heart failure. β-Blocker therapy for stable chronic heart failure patients has been shown convincingly to improve the outcome of heart failure patients, and should now be part of standard management. The use of centrally acting inhibitors of the SNS is an intriguing though not yet proven possibility.

References

1. Chidsey CA, Braunwald E, Morrow AG. Catecholamine excretion and cardiac stores of noradrenaline in congestive heart failure. *Am J Med* 1965; **39**: 442–451.

2. Thomas JA, Marks BH. Plasma noradrenaline in congestive heart failure. *Am J Cardiol* 1978; **41**: 233–243.

3. Levine TB, Francis GS, Goldsmith SR et al. Activity of the sympathetic nervous system and renin–angiotensin system assessed by plasma hormone levels and their relation to hemodynamic abnormalities in congestive heart failure. *Am J Cardiol* 1982; **49**: 1659–1666.

4. Francis GS, Satoh P, Goldsmith SR, Cohn JN. Conjugated plasma norepinephrine in patients with congestive heart failure. *Clin Res* 1982; **30**: 708A.

5. Packer M. Is activation of the sympathetic nervous system beneficial or detrimental to the patients with chronic heart failure? Lessons learned from clinical trials with beta-adrenergic agonists and antagonists. *J Cardiovasc Pharmacol* 1989; **14**: S38–S43.

6. Kaye DM, Lefkovits J, Jennings GL et al. Adverse consequences of high sympathetic nervous activity in the failing human heart. *J Am Coll Cardiol* 1995; **26**: 1257–1263.

7. Cohn JN, Levine TB, Olivari MT et al. Plasma norepinephrine as a guide to prognosis in patients with chronic congestive heart failure. *N Engl J Med* 1984; **311**: 819–823.

8. Leimbach WN, Wallin BG, Victor RG et al. Direct evidence from intraneural recordings for increased central sympathetic outflow in patients with heart failure. *Circulation* 1986; **73**: 913–919.

9. Ferguson DW, Berg WJ, Sanders JS. Clinical and haemodynamic correlates of sympathetic nerve activity in normal humans and patients with heart failure: evidence from direct microneurographic recordings. *J Am Coll Cardiol* 1990; **16**: 1125–1134.

10. Kienkle MG, Ferguson DW, Birkett CL et al. Clinical, haemodynamic and sympathetic neural correlates of heart rate variability in congestive heart failure. *Am J Cardiol* 1992; **69**: 761–767.

11. Esler M, Jennings G, Korner P et al. Assessment of human sympathetic nervous

system activity from measurements of norepinephrine turnover. *Hypertension* 1988; 11: 3–20.

12. Eckberg DL, Drabinsky M, Braunwald E. Defective parasympathetic control in patients with heart disease. *N Engl J Med* 1971; 285: 877–883.

13. Binkley PF, Nunziata E, Haas GJ et al. Parasympathetic withdrawal is an integral component of autonomic imbalance in congestive heart failure: demonstration in human subjects and verification in a paced canine model of ventricular failure. *J Am Coll Cardiol* 1991; 18: 464–472.

14. Francis GS, Goldsmith SR, Levine TB et al. The neurohumoral axis in congestive heart failure. *Ann Intern Med* 1984; 101: 377.

15. The SOLVD Investigators. Effect of enalapril on survival in patients with reduced left ventricular ejection fractions and congestive heart failure. *N Engl J Med* 1992; 325: 293–302.

16. Swedberg K, IdanpaanHeikkila U, Remes J et al. Effects of enalapril on mortality in severe congestive heart failure. Results of the Cooperative North Scandinavian Enalapril Survival Study (CONSENSUS). *N Engl J Med* 1987; 316: 1429–1435.

17. Francis GS, Cohn JN, Johnson G et al. Plasma norepinephrine, plasma renin activity, and congestive heart failure: relations to survival and the effects of therapy in V-HeFT II. *Circulation* 1993; 87: V140–V148.

18. Cohn JN, Johnson G, Ziesche S et al. A comparison of enalapril with hydralazine-isosorbide dinitrate in the treatment of chronic congestive heart failure. *N Engl J Med* 1991; 325: 303–310.

19. Pitt B, Zannad F, Remme WJ et al. The effect of spironolactone on morbidity and mortality in patients with severe heart failure. *N Engl J Med* 1999; 341: 709–717.

20. O'Connor CM, Gattis WA, Uretsky BF et al. Continuous intravenous dobutamine is associated with an increased risk of death in patients with advanced heart failure: insights from the Flolan International Randomized Survival Trial (FIRST). *Am Heart J* 1999; 138: 78–86.

21. Lang CC, Stein CM, Nelson RA et al. Sympathoinhibitory response to clonidine is blunted in patients with heart failure. *Hypertension* 1997; 30: 392–397.

22. The Xamoterol in Severe Heart Failure Study Group. Xamoterol in severe heart failure. *Lancet* 1990; 336: 1–6.

23. Maskin CS, Forman R, Klein NA et al. Long-term amrinone therapy in patients with severe heart failure: drug dependent haemodynamic benefits despite progression of the disease. *Am J Med* 1982; 72: 113–118.

24. Baim DS, McDowell AV, Cherniles J et al. Evaluation of a new bipyridine inotropic agent—milrinone—in patients with severe congestive cardiac failure. *N Engl J Med* 1983; 309: 748–756.

25. Petein M, Levine TB, Cohn JN. Persistent hemodynamic effects without long-term clinical benefits in response to oral piroximone (MDL 19,205) in patients with congestive heart failure. *Circulation* 1986; 73: III-230–III-236.

26. Shah PK, Amin DK, Hilse S et al. Inotropic therapy for refractory congestive heart failure with oral fenoximone (MDL 17,043): Poor long-term results despite early haemodynamic and clinical improvement. *Circulation* 1985; 71: 326–331.

27. Liang CS, Sherman LG, Doherty JU et al. Sustained improvement in patients with

congestive heart failure after short-term infusion of dobutamine. *Circulation* 1984; **69**: 113–119.

28. Packer M, Leier CV. Survival in congestive heart failure during treatment with drugs with positive inotropic actions. *Circulation* 1987; **75** (Suppl IV): IV-55–IV-63.

29. Shah PK, Amin DK, Horn E. Adverse clinical and haemodynamic effects of oral levodopa in chronic congestive cardiac failure. *Am Heart J* 1985; **110**: 488–489.

30. Cohn JN, Goldstein SO, Greenberg BH et al. A dose-dependent increase in mortality with vesnarinone among patients with severe heart failure. *N Engl J Med* 1998; **339**: 1810–1816.

31. Franciosa JA, Schwartz DE. Acute hemodynamic effects of norepinephrine inhibition in patients with severe chronic congestive heart failure. *J Am Coll Cardiol* 1989; **14**: 624–630.

32. Screiber R, Maier PT, Gunnar RM, Loeb HS. Haemodynamic improvement following a single oral dose of phentolamine: administration in patients with chronic low output cardiac failure. *Chest* 1976; **76**: 571–575.

33. Kovick RB, Tillisch JH, Berens SC et al. Vasodilator therapy for chronic left ventricular failure. *Circulation* 1976; **53**: 322–328.

34. Miller RR, Awan NA, Maxwell KS, Mason DT. Sustained reduction of cardiac impedance and preload in congestive heart failure with the antihypertensive vasodilator prazosin. *N Engl J Med* 1977; **297**: 303–307.

35. Awan NA, Hermanovich J, Whitcomb C et al. Cardiocirculatory effects of afterload reduction with oral trimazosin in severe congestive cardiac failure. *Am J Cardiol* 1979; **44**: 126–131.

36. Markham RV, Corbett JR, Gilmore A et al. Efficacy of prazosin in the management of chronic congestive cardiac failure: a 6-month randomized, double-blind, placebo-controlled study. *Am J Cardiol* 1983; **51**: 1346–1352.

37. Packer M, Meller J, Gorlin R, Herman MV. Haemodynamic and clinical tachyphylaxis to prazosin-mediated afterload reduction in severe chronic congestive heart failure. *Circulation* 1979; **59**: 531–539.

38. Packer M, Medina N, Yushak M. Comparative hemodynamic and clinical effects of long-term treatment with prazosin and captopril for severe chronic congestive heart failure secondary to coronary artery disease or idiopathic dilated cardiomyopathy. *Am J Cardiol* 1986; **57**: 1323–1327.

39. Colucci WS, Williams GH, Braunwald E. Increased plasma norepinephrine levels during prazosin therapy for severe congestive heart failure. *Ann Intern Med* 1980; **93**: 452–453.

40. Stein L, Henry DP, Weinberger MH. Increase in plasma norepinephrine during prazosin therapy for chronic congestive heart failure. *Am J Med* 1981; **70**: 825–832.

41. ALLHAT Collaborative Research Group. Major cardiovascular events in hypertensive patients randomized to doxazosin vs chlorthalidone: the antihypertensive and lipid-lowering treatment to prevent heart attack trial (ALLHAT). *J Am Med Assoc* 2000; **283**: 1967–1975.

42. Waagstein F, Hjalmarson A, Varnauskas E, Waalentin I. Effect of chronic beta-adrenergic receptor blockade in congestive cardiomyopathy. *Br Heart J* 1975; **37**: 1022–1036.

43. Waagstein F, Bristow MR, Swedberg K et al. Beneficial effects of metoprolol in idiopathic

dilated cardiomyopathy. *Lancet* 1993; **342**: 1441–1446.

44. CIBIS investigators. A randomized trial of beta-blockade in heart failure. The Cardiac Insufficiency Bisoprolol Study. *Circulation* 1994; **90**: 1765–1773.

45. Packer M, Bristow MR, Cohn JN et al. The effect of carvedilol on morbidity and mortality in patients with chronic heart failure. *N Engl J Med* 1996; **334**: 1349–1355.

46. Colucci WS, Packer M, Bristow MR et al. Carvedilol inhibits clinical progression in patients with mild symptoms of heart failure. *Circulation* 1996; **94**: 2800–2806.

47. Packer M, Colucci WS, Sackner Bernstein JD et al. Double-blind, placebo-controlled study of the effects of carvedilol in patients with moderate to severe heart failure: the PRECISE trial. *Circulation* 1996; **94**: 2793–2799.

48. Bristow MR, Gilbert EM, Abraham WT et al. Carvedilol produces dose-related improvements in left ventricular function and survival in subjects with chronic heart failure. *Circulation* 1996; **94**: 2807–2816.

49. Cohn J, Fowler MB, Bristow MR et al. Safety and efficacy of carvedilol in severe heart failure. The US carvedilol heart failure study group. *J Cardiac Failure* 1997; **3**: 173–179.

50. Australia–New Zealand Heart Failure Research Collaborative Group. Effects of carvedilol, a vasodilator beta-blocker, in patients with congestive heart failure due to ischaemic heart disease. *Circulation* 1995; **92**: 1499–1506.

51. CIBIS II investigators. The cardiac insufficiency bisoprolol study II (CIBIS-II): a randomised trial. *Lancet* 2000; **353**: 9–13.

52. Pollock SG, Lystash J, Tedesco C et al. Usefulness of bucindolol in congestive heart failure. *Am J Cardiol* 1990; **66**: 603–607.

53. Bristow MR, O'Connell JB, Gilbert EM et al. Dose–response of chronic beta-blocker treatment in heart failure from either idiopathic dilated or ischemic cardiomyopathy. *Circulation* 1994; **89**: 1632–1642.

54. Woodley SL, Gilbert EM, Anderson JL et al. Beta-blockade with bucindolol in heart failure caused by ischemic versus idiopathic dilated cardiomyopathy. *Circulation* 1991; **84**: 2426–2441.

55. *The Beta-blocker Evaluation Survival Study (BEST)*. Anaheim, CA: American Heart Association, 1999.

56. Witte J, Thackray S, Banerjee T et al. Update of ELITE-II, BEST, CHAMP, and IMPRESS clinical trials in heart failure. *Eur J Heart Failure* 2000; **2**: 107–112.

57. Hjalmarson A, Goldstein S, Fagerberg B et al. Effects of controlled-release metoprolol on total mortality, hospitalizations, and well-being in patients with heart failure: the Metoprolol CR/XL Randomized Intervention Trial in congestive heart failure (MERIT-HF). *J Am Med Assoc* 2000; **283**: 1295–1302.

58. Imperato McGinley J, Gautier T, Ehlers K et al. Reversibility of catecholamine-induced dilated cardiomyopathy in a child with a phaeochromocytoma. *N Engl J Med* 1987; **316**: 793–797.

59. Mann DL, Cooper G. Propranolol prevents the myopathic effects of catecholamines in vitro: implications for patients with congestive heart failure. *Circulation* 1988; **78** (Suppl II): II–576 (abstract).

60. Waagstein F, Caidahl K, Wallentin I et al. Long-term beta-blockade in dilated cardiomyopathy: effects of short- and long-term metoprolol treatment followed by withdrawal and readministration of metoprolol. *Circulation* 1989; **80**: 551–563.

61. Cleland JGF, Dargie HJ. Arrhythmias, catecholamines and electrolytes. *Am J Cardiol* 1988; **62**: 55A–59A.

62. Holmer SR, Hense H-W, Danser AHJ et al. Beta adrenergic blockers lower renin in patients treated with ACE inhibitors and diuretics. *Heart* 1998; **80**: 45–48.

63. Palatini P, Julius S. Heart rate and the cardiovascular risk. *J Hypertens* 1996; **15**: 3–17.

64. Kristal BE, Silber H, Harari G, Froom P. The association of resting heart rate with cardiovascular, cancer and all-cause mortality. *Eur Heart J* 2000; **21**: 116–124.

65. Eichhorn EJ, Bristow MR. Practical guidelines for the initiation of beta-adrenergic blockade in patients with chronic heart failure. *Am J Cardiol* 1997; **79**: 794–798.

66. MacDonald PS, Keogh AM, Aboyoun CL et al. Tolerability and efficacy of carvedilol in patients with New York Heart Association Class IV heart failure. *J Am Coll Cardiol* 1999; **33**: 924–931.

67. Kukin ML, Mannino MM, Freudenberger RS et al. Hemodynamic comparison of twice daily metoprolol tartrate with once daily metoprolol succinate in congestive heart failure. *J Am Coll Cardiol* 2000; **35**: 45–50.

68. Manolis AJ, Olympios C, Sifaki M et al. Suppressing sympathetic activation in congestive heart failure: a new therapeutic strategy. *Hypertension* 1995; **26**: 719–724.

69. Giles TD, Manolis A, Gavras I, Gavras H. Clonidine and heart failure [1]. *Hypertension* 1996; **27**: 1187–1188.

70. Manolis AJ, Olympios C, Sifaki M et al. Combined sympathetic suppression and angiotensin-converting enzyme inhibition in congestive heart failure. *Hypertension* 1997; **29**: 525–530.

71. Hermiller JB, Magorien RD, Leithe ME et al. Clonidine in congestive heart failure: a vasodilator with negative inotropic effects. *Am J Cardiol* 1983; **51**: 791–795.

72. Van Der Geest S, Van Wijk RB, Donker AJM. Clonidine withdrawal syndrome in a patient with heart failure. *Crit Care Med* 1985; **13**: 444–445.

73. Reid JL, Panfilov V, MacPhee G, Elliott HL. Clinical pharmacology of drugs acting on imidazoline and adrenergic receptors studies with clonidine, moxonidine, rilmenidine, and atenolol. *Ann NY Acad Sci* 1995; **763**: 673–678.

74. Van Zweiten PA. Central imidazoline receptors as a target for centrally acting antihypertensive drugs. *Pharm World Sci* 1995; **17**: 186–190.

75. Reis DJ. Neurons and receptors in the rostroventrolateral medulla mediating the antihypertensive actions of drugs acting at imidazoline receptors. *J Cardiovasc Pharmacol* 1996; **27**: S11–S18.

76. Prichard BNC. Clinical experience with moxonidine. *Cardiovasc Drugs Ther* 1994; **8**: 49–58.

77. Webster J, Koch HF. Aspects of tolerability of centrally acting antihypertensive drugs. *J Cardiovasc Pharmacol* 1996; **27**: S49–S54.

78. JuulMoller S, Swedberg K, Dickstein K, McNay J. Moxonidine improves heart rate variability in patients with heart failure. *J Am Coll Cardiol* 1997; **29**: 996.

79. Girgis I, Chakko S, de Marchena E et al. Effect of clonidine on heart rate variability in congestive heart failure. *Am J Cardiol* 1998; **82**: 335–337.

80. Mitrovic V, Strasser R, Walenta R et al. Haemodynamic and neurohormonal effects of

a single oral dose of the imidazoline I_1 receptor agonist moxonidine in patients with idiopathic dilated cardiomyopathy and heart failure. *Eur J Clin Res* 1996; **8:** 149–161.

81. Dickstein K, Manhenke C, Aarsland T et al. Acute hemodynamic and neurohormonal effects of moxonidine in congestive heart failure secondary to ischaemic or idiopathic dilated cardiomyopathy. *Am J Cardiol* 1999; **83:** 1638–1644.

82. Wenzel RR, Qui S, Speiker L et al. Moxonidine decreases both cardiac and peripheral sympathetic activity in healthy volunteers. *Kidney Blood Press Res* 1996; **19:** 63 (abstract).

83. Azevedo ER, Newton GE, Parker JD. Cardiac and systemic sympathetic activity in response to clonidine in human heart failure. *J Am Coll Cardiol* 1999; **33:** 186–191.

84. Swedberg K, Bergh C-H, Dickstein K et al. The effects of moxonidine, a novel imidazoline, on plasma norepinephrine in patients with congestive heart failure. *J Am Coll Cardiol* 2000; **35:** 398–404.

85. Sustained Release Moxonidine for Congestive Heart Failure: the MOXCON study. *3rd International Heart Failure Meeting*, European Society of Cardiology, Gothenberg, 1999.

86. Hampton JR, Van VD, Kleber FX et al. Randomised study of effect of ibopramine on survival in patients with advanced severe heart failure. *Lancet* 1997; **349:** 971–977.

87. Cowley AJ, Skene AM. Treatment of severe heart failure: quantity or quality of life? A trial of enoximone. Enoximone investigators. *Br Heart J* 1994; **72:** 226–230.

88. Cowley AJ, McEntegart DJ, Hampton JR et al. Long-term evaluation of treatment for chronic heart failure: a 1 year comparative trial of flosequinan and captopril. *Cardiovasc Drugs Ther* 1994; **8:** 829–836.

89. Lechat P, Jaillon P, Fontaine ML et al. A randomized trial of beta-blockade in heart failure: The Cardiac Insufficiency Bisoprolol Study (CIBIS). *Circulation* 1994; **90:** 1765–1773.

90. Kirlin PC, Das S, Grekin R et al. Sympathetic inhibition with methyldopa in heart failure. *J Cardiovasc Pharmacol* 1986; **8:** 1092–1100.

91. Olivari MT, Levine TB, Cohn JN. Acute hemodynamic and hormonal effects of central versus peripheral sympathetic inhibition in patients with congestive heart failure. *J Cardiovasc Pharmacol* 1986; **8:** 973–977.

92. Giles TD, Thomas MG, Sander GE, Quiroz AC. Central alpha-adrenergic agonists in chronic heart failure and ischemic heart disease. *J Cardiovasc Pharmacol* 1985; **7:** S51–S55.

93. Good AP, Unverferth DV, Leier CV. Hemodynamic responses to different levels of alpha-adrenergic interruption in congestive heart failure. *Cardiovasc Drugs Ther* 1988; **1:** 529–534.

94. Magorien RD, Hermiller JB, Unverferth DV, Leier CV. Regional hemodynamic effects of clonidine in congestive heart failure. *J Cardiovasc Pharmacol* 1985; **7:** 91–96.

95. Lang CC, Rayos GH, Chomsky DB et al. Effect of sympathoinhibition on exercise performance in patients with heart failure. *Circulation* 1997; **96:** 238–245.

96. Swedberg K, Waagstein F, Dickstein K et al. Moxonidine, a centrally acting sympathetic inhibitor, causes sustained reduction of plasma norepinephrine in heart failure patients. *J Am Coll Cardiol* 1997; **29:** 7625.

97. Dickstein K, Kopp U, Manhenke C et al. The hemodynamic and neurohormonal effects of moxonidine, a sympathetic inhibitor. *J Am Coll Cardiol* 1997; **29**: 7275.

98. Coats AJS, Adamopoulos S, Radaelli A et al. Controlled trial of physical training in chronic heart failure: exercise performance, hemodynamics, ventilation, and autonomic function. *Circulation* 1992; **85**: 2119–2131.

99. Ribner HS, Plucinski DA, Hseieh AM et al. Acute effects of digoxin on total systemic vascular resistance in congestive heart failure due to dilated cardiomyopathy. *Am J Cardiol* 1985; **56**: 896–904.

100. Ferguson DW, Berg WJ, Saunders JS et al. Sympathoinhibitory responses to digitalis glycosides in heart failure patients. *Circulation* 1989; **80**: 65–77.

Other treatment strategies: a non-pharmacological approach

Colin Berry

9

Introduction

Whilst drug treatments remain the key therapy in the management of chronic heart failure, non-pharmacological interventions are being increasingly viewed as useful adjunctive measures. Non-pharmacological strategies may be effective in both attenuating disease progression and improving symptoms, as may be the case with exercise training. The ethos of non-drug interventions embraces the philosophy of treating the whole patient and addressing dietary, psychological, sexual and sociological needs. One important advance toward achieving these aims has been through the development of nurse-led community management programmes. Furthermore, non-pharmacological strategies may also be cost-effective. In this chapter, developments in the field of non-pharmacological interventions in chronic heart failure are reviewed.

Exercise training

Traditionally, rest was recommended for patients with chronic heart failure. However, there is a growing body of evidence to support the beneficial effects of exercise therapy in heart failure patients. Should we now reconsider our advice to heart failure patients?

Skeletal muscle in heart failure

All body systems, including skeletal muscle, are involved in the development of the heart failure syndrome. Skeletal muscle dysfunction comprises muscle fibre atrophy,[1] shift in fibre type to a higher proportion of anaerobic type IIb fibres, impaired oxidative capacity at rest and during exercise,[2] impaired blood flow[3] and metaboreceptor dysfunction.[4] The metaboreceptors are sensitive to work performed by skeletal muscle. In part they are responsible for the ventilatory response to exercise and are more active than usual in patients with heart failure. Skeletal muscle has reduced strength,[5,6] and fatigues early.[7] Overall, impaired skeletal muscle function contributes to exercise intolerance[8] and is related to the severity of heart failure.[9]

The cause of the skeletal myopathy is not clear. Physical deconditioning may contribute to skeletal muscle dysfunction.[10] Sympathetic and cytokine activation are pathophysiological processes that contribute to abnormal skeletal muscle metabolism.[11] There is a general metabolic change in heart failure in favour of catabolic over anabolic processes,[12] including insulin and growth hormone resistance, and rise in the ratio of catabolic to anabolic

steroids. These changes might contribute to muscle changes.

The training response

Evidence from clinical studies now suggests that exercise training improves skeletal muscle dysfunction in patients with heart failure. In an early study, cycle training increased the threshold for anaerobic metabolism and enhanced exercise endurance.[13] Subsequently, a multitude of studies in small numbers of selected patients have shown that training induces an improvement of about 20% in peak aerobic capacity in heart failure (*Table 9.1*).

Following training, there are increases in both exercise duration at fixed workloads[13] and the distance covered in a 6-minute walk test.[14,15]

Exercise training can also improve symptoms and quality of life in heart failure patients.[13,16–18] The benefits of endurance training have compared favourably with those of angiotensin converting enzyme (ACE) inhibitor treatment.[19] The ventilatory response to exercise is reduced by training,[20] and there are improvements in indices of sympathetic overactivity.[16,21]

Mechanisms of benefit

Skeletal muscle metabolism is altered by training; in patients who performed a

Table 9.1
Training regimes and improvement in peak exercise capacity seen in selected exercise training studies in chronic heart failure

First author	Age of patients (years)	n	Study design	Type of training	Frequency	Duration	↑Peak Vo_2 (%)
Sullivan[13]	54 (10)	24	All trained	Cycling, walking	60 min, 3–5/week	16–24 weeks	23
Coats[18,31]	61.8 ± 1.5	17	Crossover	Cycling	20 min, 5/week	8 weeks	18
Meyer[73]	52 ± 2	18	Crossover	Cycling, walking (interval*)	45 min, 11/week	3 weeks	20
Kiilavuori[74]	52 (8)	27	Randomized	Walking, cycling	30 min, 3/week	5 months	12
		12	Trained				
Keteyian[75]	56 (11)	40	Randomized	Treadmill, cycling, rowing	45 min, 3/week	24 weeks	16
		21	Trained				
Kavanagh[15]	62 (6)	17	Trained	Walking	10–21 km/week	52 weeks	17
Hambrecht[25]	51 (10)	22	Randomized	Cycling	40 min daily	6 months	33
		12	Trained				
Belardinelli[39]	57 (6)	27	18 Trained, 9 matched controls	Cycling	30 min, 3/week	8 weeks	17
Demopoulos[38]	61 ± 2	16	All trained	Cycling	60 min, 4/week	12 weeks	22

↑ Peak Vo_2 is the percentage increase in peak oxygen consumption (ml/kg per minute) seen after training.
*Interval training is characterized by repeated short bursts of exercise, with recovery periods in between.

programme of isolated forearm handgrip exercises, there was improved metabolic performance, and an increase in exercise capacity independent of any change in blood flow, muscle mass or VO_2max.[22,23] Adamopoulos et al demonstrated a decrease in phosphocreatine depletion and a shortening in the recovery time of phosphocreatine following exercise with training.[24] The results of forearm training are similar, with an improved pH response to exercise.[25] In an animal model, the skeletal muscle metabolic benefits were shown to be independent of changes in muscle bulk.[26] Hambrecht et al have demonstrated changes to muscle structure with exercise training, and increases in mitochondrial density.[27,28] These changes were independent of systemic haemodynamic training effects.

Exercise training can, therefore, result in enhanced metabolic and oxidative efficiency within skeletal muscle, independent of other exercise-related physiological changes.

Exercising skeletal muscle increases ventilation via activation of peripheral neuromuscular reflexes.[29] In patients with chronic heart failure, overactivity of this physiological reflex may cause an increase in the ventilatory response to exercise,[30] leading to symptoms of breathlessness. Training, in the form of handgrip exercise, reduced the enhanced ergoreflex drive to ventilation.[31] The respiratory muscle is affected by the same changes as skeletal muscle more generally, and specific respiratory muscle training resulted in

objective improvement in ventilation and exercise capacity.[32]

Some (but not all) studies have shown improvements in central haemodynamics[33] after exercise training. This seems unlikely to be a major contributor to the training effect; central haemodynamic variables are not a strong determinant of symptoms or exercise capacity in heart failure patients. Patients with chronic heart failure usually have normal submaximal cardiac output responses[34,35] and it is difficult to see how normal responses could be improved. Wilson et al reported that training benefits were restricted to those patients with normal haemodynamic responses[36] and that those patients with subnormal responses before a training programme were unlikely to benefit.

Exercise causes changes in peripheral and central blood flow. In particular, there is enhanced perfusion of exercising skeletal muscle, the heart and the kidney. However, in heart failure patients, the normal increase in blood flow within exercising skeletal muscle is attenuated.[37] Furthermore, exercise training is also associated with improved endothelium-dependent increases in forearm blood flow in heart failure.[38]

Exercise training modalities in heart failure

The ideal training regimen is not yet clear. The European Heart Failure Training Group reviewed 134 patients from six centres,[17] and described a wide variety of different training protocols. Cycle ergometer training was commonest, usually 4–5 times per week, for 20 minutes at 70–80% of peak heart rate in association with warm-up and cool-down periods. Others followed calisthenic (light gymnastic) exercises. The majority of the group (69.4%) were home based, whereas 19.4% trained only in hospital and 11.2% followed a combined training programme. The duration of training ranged from 6 to 16 weeks.

The intensity of training required is also unclear. Typically, training programmes are at around 70% of maximal exercise capacity. Two studies have demonstrated positive effects with far lower levels of exertion,[39,40] and this lighter training may make training a more realistic prospect for more frail patients.

Importantly, follow-up data on morbidity and mortality are required before this therapy could be routinely prescribed. One recent single-centre controlled study of exercise rehabilitation in 99 heart failure patients reported improvements in exercise capacity, quality of life, hospital readmissions and all-cause mortality after 14 months' therapy and after a further 12 months' follow-up,[18] but this study was too small to be the basis for wider recommendations.

There have been concerns about the safety of exercise training since the publication of early work by Judgutt et al.[41] In this small,

uncontrolled study, patients trained shortly after an anterior infarct developed an increase in left ventricular size and lack of co-ordination. However, subsequent studies have shown no difference in left ventricular function between trained patients and a control group.[42,43] Exercise is safe, however, only in selected patients. Patients with decompensated chronic heart failure, unstable angina, documented ventricular arrhythmia and obstructive valve disease should not be included in exercise training programmes. At present, exercise training programmes should be initiated by hospital-based physicians in co-ordination with a cardiac rehabilitation programme. Future targets include the development of exercise programmes in the community.

A calmer approach to training may be yoga. In one controlled study, respiratory training to decrease respiratory rate to about 6 breaths per minute over a 1-month period was shown to improve resting arterial oxygen saturation, minute ventilation, peak oxygen consumption and exercise capacity.[44]

Nutrition and dietary interventions

Salt restriction

Heart failure is characterized by sodium and water retention, and standard advice for many years used to be to follow a low-salt diet. The availability of powerful loop diuretics has meant that dietary advice has rather slipped into the background. Salt (NaCl) intake in a typical Western diet is approximately 10 g per day, which is equivalent to 17.1 mmol (4 g) of sodium. In healthy subjects, a 50% reduction in salt intake will effect a 1–1.5-litre decrease in extracellular fluid volume.[45] No such data are available in heart failure patients. Salt restriction is advocated on an empirical basis, in the absence of evidence from properly conducted trials. Very low dietary salt intake (less than 2 g per day) is unpalatable and compliance is poor. Current dietary recommendations for patients with chronic heart failure should include moderation of salt intake. Dietary salt is found in the greatest proportion in processed meats, fish, tinned foods, savouries and preserves. Caution is advised when using salt substitutes as some are rich in potassium and, when taken in large quantities with an ACE inhibitor, can lead to hyperkalaemia.[46]

Fluid restriction

Fluid balance is of paramount importance in the management of heart failure. In mild disease, formal fluid restriction is usually not necessary, but patients should be advised to moderate their daily fluid intake. Fluid balance may be accurately measured by recording daily body weight which can be done at home with standard weighing scales (1 l of water = 1 kg body weight).

With more severe heart failure, particularly where more than 80 mg a day of frusemide (or its equivalent) are necessary, a patient should limit daily fluid volume to 1.5–2 litres. More strict limits, to 1.5 litres per day or less, may be helpful in managing patients who develop hyponatraemia, and in those who develop 'diuretic resistance'. Such restriction can lead to severe thirst, and, where necessary, suggests that the immediate prognosis is very poor.

Calorie intake

Dietary caloric intake must be appropriate to the individual patient. Routine clinical assessment of the heart failure patient should include both diet and weight history.

Obesity is a risk factor for hypertension and is associated with dyslipidaemia. Increased waist circumference and waist-to-hip ratio are related to insulin resistance and diabetes mellitus.[47] In heart failure, obesity is more prevalent at the time of diagnosis and in those with mild disease, than in patients with severe heart failure. Weight reduction can help with symptoms of breathlessness and fatigue, and may be best obtained through a calorie-controlled diet coupled to regular daily exercise.

Weight loss and cardiac cachexia may occur, particularly as the disease progresses. Clinically important weight loss (e.g. loss of 7.5% of dry body weight over 6 months) is an adverse prognostic feature.[48] The reasons for cachexia are complex and not well understood. Patients with heart failure may have an increased basal metabolic rate, and have a generalized imbalance between catabolic and anabolic metabolic processes.[12] This manifests as insulin resistance, growth hormone resistance and activation of cytokines (such as tumour necrosis factor). Malnutrition can also be a problem; the elderly, in particular, may have a poor diet and are more prone to anorexia. Iatrogenic factors, such as digoxin-induced nausea, are potentially remediable causes. Malabsorption, particularly of dietary fats may also contribute to malnutrition and is associated with cachexia in heart failure patients.[49]

Caloric intake is an important consideration in heart failure. Dietary advice should be given in conjunction with a dietitian. The only randomized placebo-controlled trial of a dietary intervention (high protein energy diet) did not show any clinical benefit.[50] However, in this study only two patients fulfilled standard criteria for malnutrition and the small numbers in each group were such that this study was underpowered to detect differences between the two groups. Patients with cachexia should have a high-energy diet with a high content of both carbohydrate and protein. They should also be advised to maintain a minimum recommended daily energy intake of 2800 kCal.

Vitamin intake

In some studies, increased dietary intake of antioxidants such as vitamin C and vitamin E in patients with ischaemic heart disease has been associated with beneficial effects.[51,52] Heart failure is characterized by oxidant stress.[53] Endothelial dysfunction has been demonstrated in vivo in heart failure patients[54,55] and vascular oxidant stress is thought to contribute to impaired endothelial function in heart failure. It might be thought that supplementation with vitamins C and E should be beneficial, but there is no definitive evidence in support of this hypothesis. The recent publication of the HOPE study has dampened enthusiasm for vitamin E therapy.[56]

Thiamine deficiency is common in chronic heart failure, particularly in the elderly[57] and in patients who take high doses of loop diuretics.[58] In one intervention study in heart failure patients taking frusemide, thiamine supplementation was associated with improved left ventricular ejection fraction.[59]

Other dietary supplements are being evaluated. Oral proprionyl-L-carnitine has in some studies shown improved exercise tolerance (but not haemodynamic variables) in patients with chronic heart failure,[60] and in some studies, creatine supplementation has been shown to improve skeletal muscle function.[61] This is an area of much research interest at present, and no clear recommendations can yet be made.

Alcohol intake

Alcohol causes acute peripheral vasodilatation and may also impair myocardial contractility. Alcohol is directly implicated in the aetiology of dilated cardiomyopathy. In patients with alcoholic cardiomyopathy, abstinence from alcohol is associated with an improvement in symptoms and signs of heart failure and in left ventricular ejection fraction.[62]

Alcohol is not contraindicated in heart failure due to other causes and, indeed, may be associated with a better outcome.[63]

Cigarette smoking

Smoking, vascular dysfunction and cardiovascular disease are integrally related. Although there is little direct evidence on prognosis in heart failure per se, patients should be encouraged to give up smoking. Cigarette smoking causes impaired endothelium-dependant vasorelaxation and vasospasm in heart failure patients.[64] The risk of reinfarction after a heart attack is halved if the patient stops smoking.

The patient should be positively encouraged on how to stop smoking. Nicotine therapy is a useful tool to help patients stop smoking.[65] Nicotine patches may be safely used by patients with stable angina or 4 weeks after myocardial infarction.[66] Nicotine treatment should be for no longer than 6 weeks in duration. The dose of nicotine should be titrated according to the number of cigarettes smoked (2 mg daily for <15 cigarettes per day; 4 mg for 4 weeks for >15 cigarettes per day).

A 'quitting programme' is one way of formalizing the intention to stop smoking. A proposed strategy would be:

1. Set a quit date.
2. Involve family members and friends, in particular to ensure that others in the household refrain from smoking in the presence of the patient.
3. Avoid places where the patient usually buys or smokes cigarettes.
4. Arrange appointments with the primary care team for encouragement and the setting of calendar targets.

Psychological aspects

Heart failure may cause significant problems in relation to a patient's mental health. Morbidity, poor quality of life and, in some cases, low income contribute to negative emotions and depression. This in itself increases the mortality rate in patients with coronary artery disease,[67] and antidepressant therapy can be valuable in individual patients. Training on how to relax may be associated with beneficial effects.[68]

Education

Patients can make a significant contribution to their own management. Education to detect early signs of fluid retention, regulation of fluid intake, optimal drug compliance, awareness of drug side-effects, appropriate diet and the need for exercise are just some of the important issues regarding patients and their health. Patients should also be advised on monitoring their weight, their daily fluid intake and on how to modify their diuretic dose according to fluctuations in body weight. Similarly, involvement of family members and friends in this process is important.

Drug compliance

Poor compliance with medication is a feature of patients with chronic disease. Patients who adhere poorly to medication are more prone to episodes of clinical deterioration and rehospitalization.[69] Measures to optimize patient compliance with prescribed medication include nurse-led intervention studies and community-based pharmacy counselling. In one such programme, a pharmacist-led programme using pill counts produced a reduction in symptoms and an increase in exercise capacity during a 6-minute walk.[70]

Nurse-led community-based multidisciplinary programmes

Factors implicated in readmission to hospital with decompensated heart failure are non-compliance with medication, inability to

recognize signs of deteriorating health, recurrent chest infection and poor outpatient follow-up.[71] Furthermore, heart failure is increasingly a disease of the elderly. Nurse-based intervention studies in heart failure target these very issues, and is developing into a useful clinical tool. It is discussed in more detail in Chapter 10.

Surgical treatments and devices

A variety of surgical interventions is becoming available for the treatment of heart failure (*Table 9.2*). There is no doubt that, in individual patients with coronary artery disease, revascularization can result in dramatic reversal of left ventricular dysfunction. There are, as yet, no data from controlled studies to recommend this approach more widely. In selected patients where mitral regurgitation is prominent, mitral valve surgery (either valvuloplasty or valve replacement) at the same time as revascularization may help.

The Batista procedure has received much media attention. In this, the geometry and size of the left ventricular chamber are improved by removing a variable amount of the left ventricular myocardium from the apex of the heart to reduce chamber volume and normalize wall stress. This is an appealing concept, but in controlled clinical trials, the procedure has not lived up to its initial

Table 9.2
Surgical and device therapy for chronic heart failure now available and in development

'Conventional' surgery	Revascularization
	Mitral repair/replacement
Transplantation	Orthotopic
	Xenotransplants?
Artificial hearts	Bridge to transplant
	Long-term support?
Experimental surgery	Cardiomyoplasty
	Left ventricular reduction (Batista)
Electrophysiology	Defibrillators
	Sequential AV pacing
	Biventricular pacing

promise. Another approach has been cardiomyoplasty, using skeletal muscle (usually latissimus dorsi) to wrap the heart, then training the muscle to behave as 'myocardium' by pacing. Initial enthusiasm for this approach has also waned.

Cardiac transplantation is widely available, if limited by the availability of donor organs. The decision to transplant is an onerous one for both physician and patient. It is emphatically not a cure, and carries with it the risks of life-long immunosuppression. It may improve life expectancy, but does not restore it to normal; it may improve symptoms, but does not return the patient to normal. In making the decision to transplant, evidence of left ventricular dysfunction on its own is not enough. Some functional information is also essential. A valuable tool is exercise testing with metabolic gas exchange. Where peak oxygen consumption is greater than 14 ml/kg per minute, the prognosis is usually better with the native rather than a transplanted heart.

Xenotransplantation with pig hearts is moving closer, and offers the potential for unlimited availability of organs. Many technical problems remain, and government-imposed restrictions on transgenic animal research may delay further progress. Left ventricular assist devices (LVADs) and artificial hearts continue to be developed. These devices at present provide a bridge to transplant for selected patients, and some patients have survived with their circulation supported by an LVAD for several years. Quality of life, myocardial function and risk of death may be improved by this therapy.[72] Occasionally, patients develop sufficient recovery of myocardial function for the LVAD subsequently to be explanted.

Implantable cardiodefibrillator devices reduce mortality in patients with malignant ventricular arrhythmias and resuscitated cardiac arrest. The data so far suggest that the benefit is greatest in those patients with the worst cardiac function. Of course, sudden death is one of the commonest modes of death in heart failure, usually attributed to arrhythmia. Ongoing trials have been designed to address whether defibrillators are beneficial in an unselected heart failure population. If defibrillators are proven to confer a mortality benefit, this will have major implications for health care expenditure.

Advancing pacemaker technology also provides some symptomatic benefit for selected patients. In patients with long atrioventricular delay, and particularly in those with long QRS complexes, dual chamber pacing may reduce mitral regurgitation. Biventricular pacing (using a pacing lead in a tributary of the coronary sinus to pace the left ventricle) improves ventricular function in some patients (see Chapter 11).

References

1. Drexler H, Reide U, Munzel T et al. Alterations of skeletal muscle in chronic heart failure. *Circulation* 1992; **85**: 1751–1759.

2. Sullivan M, Green H, Cobb FR. Altered skeletal muscle metabolic response to exercise in chronic heart failure. *Circulation* 1991; **84**: 1597–1607.

3. Lejemtel TH, Maskin CS, Lucido D, Chadwick BJ. Failure to augment maximal limb blood flow in response to one-leg versus two-leg exercise in patients with severe heart failure. *Circulation* 1986; **74**: 245–251.

4. Sterns DA, Ettinger SM, Gray KS et al. Skeletal muscle metaboreceptor exercise responses are attenuated in heart failure. *Circulation* 1991; **84**: 2304–2039.

5. Volterrani M, Clark AL, Ludman PF et al. Determinants of exercise capacity in chronic heart failure. *Eur Heart J* 1994; **15**: 801–809.

6. Buller NP, Jones D, Poole-Wilson PA. Direct measurements of skeletal muscle fatigue in patients with chronic heart failure. *Br Heart J* 1991; **65**: 20–24.

7. Minotti JR, Pillay P, Chang L et al. Neurophysiological assessment of skeletal muscle fatigue in patients with congestive heart failure. *Circulation* 1992; **86**: 903–908.

8. Mancini DM, Walter G, Reichek N et al. Contribution of skeletal muscle atrophy to exercise intolerance and altered muscle metabolism in heart failure. *Circulation* 1992; **85**: 1364–1373.

9. Massie B, Conway M, Yonge R et al. Skeletal muscle metabolism in patients with congestive heart failure: relation to clinical severity and blood flow. *Circulation* 1987; **76**: 1009–1019.

10. Chati Z, Zannand F, Jeandel C et al. Physical deconditioning may be a mechanism for the skeletal muscle energy phosphate metabolism abnormalities in chronic heart failure. *Am Heart J* 1996; **131**: 560–566.

11. Packer M. Is tumour necrosis factor an important neurohormonal mechanism in chronic heart failure? *Circulation* 1995; **92**: 1379–1382.

12. Berry C, Clark AL. Catabolism in chronic heart failure. *Eur Heart J* 2000; **21**: 521–532.

13. Sullivan MJ, Higginbotham MB, Cobb FR. Exercise training in patients with chronic heart failure delays ventilatory anaerobic threshold and improves submaximal exercise tolerance. *Circulation* 1989; 79: 324–329.

14. Meyer K, Schwaibold M, Westbrook S et al. Effects of exercise training and activity restriction on 6-minute walking test performance in patients with chronic heart failure. *Am Heart J* 1997; 133: 447–453.

15. Kavanagh T, Myers MG, Baigrie RS et al. Quality of life and cardiorespiratory function in chronic heart failure: effects of 12 months' aerobic training. *Heart* 1996; 76: 42–49.

16. Coats AJS, Adampoulos S, Radeilli A et al. Controlled clinical trial of physical training in chronic heart failure. *Circulation* 1992; 85: 2119–2131.

17. European Heart Failure Training Group. Experience from controlled trials of physical training in chronic heart failure. *Eur Heart J* 1998; 19: 466–475.

18. Belardinelli R, Georgiou D, Cianci G, Purcaro A. Randomised, controlled trial of long-term moderate exercise training in chronic heart failure. *Circulation* 1999; 99: 1173–1182.

19. Meyer TE, Casadei B, Coats AJS et al. Angiotensin converting enzyme inhibitors and physical training in heart failure. *J Intern Med* 1991; 230: 407–413.

20. Davey P, Meyer T, Coats A et al. Ventilation in chronic heart failure: effects of physical training. *Br Heart J* 1992; 68: 473–477.

21. Adamopoulos S, Ponikowski P, Cerquetani E et al. Circadian patterns of heart rate variability in chronic heart failure patients: effects of training. *Eur Heart J* 1995; 16: 1380–1386.

22. Minotti JR, Johnson EC, Hudson TL et al. Training-induced skeletal muscle adaptations are independent of systemic adaptations. *J Appl Physiol* 1990; 68: 289–294.

23. Minotti JR, Johnson EC, Hudson TL et al. Skeletal muscle responses to exercise training in chronic heart failure. *J Clin Invest* 1990; 86: 751–758.

24. Adamopoulos S, Coats AJS, Brunotte F et al. Physical training improves skeletal muscle metabolic abnormalities in patients with chronic heart failure. *J Am Coll Cardiol* 1993; 23: 1101–1106.

25. Stratton JR, Dunn JF, Adamopoulos S et al. Training partially reverses skeletal muscle metabolic abnormalities during exercise in heart failure. *J Appl Physiol* 1994; 76: 1575–1582.

26. Brunotte F, Thompson CH, Adamopoulos S et al. Rat skeletal muscle metabolism in experimental heart failure: effects of physical training. *Acta Physiol Scand* 1995; 154: 439–447.

27. Hambrecht R, Niebauer J, Fiehn E et al. Physical training in patients with stable chronic heart failure: effects on cardiorespiratory fitness and ultrastructural abnormalities of leg muscles. *J Am Coll Cardiol* 1995; 25: 1239–1249.

28. Hambrecht R, Fiehn E, Yu J et al. Effects of endurance training on mitochondrial ultrastructure and fiber type distribution in skeletal muscle of patients with stable chronic heart failure. *J Am Coll Cardiol* 1997; 29: 1067–1073.

29. Piepoli M, Clark AL, Coats AJS. Muscle metaboreceptors in hemodynamic, autonomic, and ventilatory responses to exercise in men. *Am J Physiol* 1995; 269: H1428–H1436.

30. Clark AL, Poole-Wilson PA, Coats AJS. Exercise limitation in chronic heart failure: the central role of the periphery. *J Am Coll Cardiol* 1996; **28**: 1092–1102.

31. Piepoli M, Clark AL, Volterrani M et al. Contribution of muscle afferents to the hemodynamic, autonomic and ventilatory reponses to exercise in patients with chronic heart failure. *Circulation* 1996; **93**: 940–952.

32. Mancini DM, Hensen D, La Manca J et al. Benefit of selective respiratory muscle training on exercise capacity in patients with chronic congestive heart failure. *Circulation* 1995; **91**: 320–329.

33. Coats AJS, Adamopoulos S, Meyer TE et al. Effects of physical training in chronic heart failure. *Lancet* 1990; **335**: 63–66.

34. Wilson JR, Mancini DM, Dunkman WB. Exertional fatigue due to skeletal muscle dysfunction in patients with heart failure. *Circulation* 1993; **87**: 470–475.

35. Wilson JR, Rayos G, Yeoh TK, Gothard P. Dissociation between peak exercise oxygen consumption and hemodynamic dysfunction in potential heart transplantation candidates. *J Am Coll Cardiol* 1995; **26**: 429–435.

36. Wilson JR, Groves J, Rayos G. Circulatory status and response to cardiac rehabilitation in patients with heart failure. *Circulation* 1996; **94**: 1567–1572.

37. Muller AF, Batin P, Evans S et al. Regional blood flow in chronic heart failure; the reason for the lack of correlation between exercise tolerance and cardiac output? *Br Heart J* 1992; **67**: 478–481.

38. Hornig B, Maier V, Drexler H. Physical training improves endothelial function in patients with chronic heart failure. *Circulation* 1996; **93**: 201–204.

39. Demopoulos LJ, Bijou R, Fergus I et al. Exercise training in patients with severe congestive heart failure; enhancing peak aerobic capacity while minimising the increase in ventricular wall stress. *J Am Coll Cardiol* 1997; **29**: 597–603.

40. Belardinelli R, Georgiou D, Scocco V et al. Low intensity exercise training in patients with chronic heart failure. *J Am Coll Cardiol* 1995; **26**: 975–982.

41. Jugdutt BI, Michorowski BL, Kappagoda CT. Exercise training after anterior Q wave myocardial infarction: importance of left ventricular function and topography. *J Am Coll Cardiol* 1988; **12**: 362–372.

42. Gianuzzi P, Tavazzi L, Temporelli PL et al., for the EAMI study group. Long-term physical training and left ventricular remodelling after anterior myocardial infarction (EAMI) trial. *J Am Coll Cardiol* 1993; **22**: 1821–1829.

43. Ehsani AA, Miller TR, Miller TA et al. Comparison of adaptations to a 12-month exercise program and late outcome in patients with healed myocardial infarction and ejection fraction <45% and >50%. *Am J Cardiol* 1997; **79**: 1258–1260.

44. Bernardi L, Spadacini G, Bellwon J et al. Effect of breathing rate on oxygen saturation and exercise performance in chronic heart failure. *Lancet* 1998; **351**: 1308–1311.

45. Antonios TFT, MacGregor GA. Salt—more adverse effects. *Lancet* 1996; **348**: 250–251.

46. Good CB, McDermott L, McCloskey B. Diet and serum potassium in patients on ACE inhibitors. *JAMA* 1995; **274**: 538.

47. Schmidt MI, Duncan SS, Canani LH et al. Association of waist–hip ratio with diabetes-mellitus—strength and possible modifiers. *Diabetes Care* 1992; **15**: 912–914.

48. Anker S, Ponikowski P, Varney S et al. Wasting as an independent risk factor for mortality in chronic heart failure. *Lancet* 1997; **349**: 1050–1053.

49. King D, Smith ML, Chapman TJ et al. Fat malabsorption in elderly patients with cardiac cachexia. *Age Ageing* 1996; **25**: 144–149.

50. Broqvist M, Arnqvist H, Dahlstrom U et al. Nutritional assessment and muscle energy metabolism in severe chronic congestive heart failure—effects of long-term dietary supplementation. *Eur Heart J* 1994; **15**: 1641–1650.

51. Kush LH, Folsom AR, Prineas RJ et al. Dietary antioxidant vitamins and death from coronary heart disease in postmenopausal women. *N Engl J Med* 1996; **334**: 1156–1162.

52. Stephens NG, Parsons A, Schofield PM et al. Randomised controlled trial of vitamin E in patients with coronary disease: Cambridge Heart Antioxidant Study (CHAOS). *Lancet* 1996; **347**: 781–786.

53. McMurray J, Chopra M, Abdullah I et al. Evidence of oxidative stress in chronic heart failure in humans. *Eur Heart J* 1993; **14**: 1493–1498.

54. Drexler H, Hayoz D, Munzel T et al. Endothelial function in chronic congestive heart failure. *Am J Cardiol* 1992; **69**: 1596–1601.

55. Kubo SH, Rector TS, Bank AJ et al. Endothelium-dependent vasodilation is attenuated in patients with heart failure. *Circulation* 1991; **84**: 1589–1596.

56. The Heart Outcomes Prevention Evaluation Study Investigators. Vitamin E supplementation and cardiovascular events in high-risk patients. *N Engl J Med* 2000; **342**: 154–160.

57. Kwok T, Falconersmith JF, Potter JF, Ives DR. Thiamine status of elderly patients with cardiac failure. *Age Aging* 1992; **21**: 67–71.

58. Seligmann H, Halikin H, Rauchfleisch S et al. Thiamine deficiency in patients with congestive heart failure receiving long term furosemide therapy—a pilot study. *Am J Med* 1991; **91**: 151–155.

59. Shimon I, Almog S, Vered Z et al. Improved left ventricular function after thiamine supplementation in patients with congestive heart failure receiving long term furosemide therapy. *Am J Med* 1995; **98**: 485–490.

60. Anand I, Chandrashekhan Y, De Giuli F et al. Acute and chronic effects of propionyl-L-carnitine on the hemodynamics, exercise capacity, and hormones in patients with congestive heart failure. *Cardiovasc Drugs Ther* 1998; **12**: 291–299.

61. Gordon A, Hultman E, Kaijser L. Creatine supplementation in chronic heart failure increases skeletal muscle creatine phosphate and muscle performance. *Cardiovasc Res* 1995; **30**: 413–418.

62. Jacob AJ, McLaren KM, Boon NA. Effects of abstinence on alcoholic heart-muscle disease. *Am J Cardiol* 1991; **68**: 805–807.

63. Cooper HA, Exner DV, Domanski MJ. Light-to-moderate alcohol consumption and prognosis in patients with left ventricular systolic dysfunction. *J Am Coll Cardiol* 2000; **35**: 1753–1759.

64. Nicolozakes AW, Binkley PF, Leier CV. Haemodynamic effects of smoking in congestive heart failure. *Am J Med Sci* 1988; **286**: 377–380.

65. Tang JL, Law M, Wald N. How effective is nicotine replacement therapy in helping people to stop smoking? *Br Med J* 1994; **308**: 21–26.

66. Silagy C, Mant D, Fowler G, Lodge M. Meta-analysis on efficacy of nicotine replacement therapies in smoking cessation. *Lancet* 1994; 343: 139–142.

67. Frasure-Smith N, Lesperance F, Talajic M. Depression and 18 month prognosis after myocardial infarction. *Circulation* 1995; 91: 999–1005.

68. Hyman RB, Feldman HR, Harris RB et al. The effects of relaxation training on clinical symptoms—a meta analysis. *Nurs Res* 1989; 38: 216–220.

69. Ghali JK, Kadakia S, Cooper R, Ferlinz J. Precipitating factors leading to decompensation of heart failure. *Ann Intern Med* 1988; 148: 2013–2016.

70. Goodyer L, Miskelly F, Milligan P. Does encouraging good compliance improve patients' clinical condition in heart failure? *Br J Clin Pract* 1995; 49: 173–176.

71. Chin MH, Goldman L. Correlates of early hospital readmission or death in patients with congestive heart failure. *Am J Cardiol* 1997; 79: 1640–1644.

72. Moskowitz AJ, Weinberg AD, Oz MC, Williams DL. Quality of life with an implanted left ventricular assist device. *Ann Thorac Surg* 1997; 64: 1764–1769.

73. Meyer K, Schwaibold M, Westbrook S et al. Effect of short-term exercise training and activity restriction on functional capacity in patients with severe chronic congestive heart failure. *Am J Cardiol* 1996; 78: 1017–1022.

74. Kiilavuori K, Sovijärvi A, Näveri H et al. Effect of physical training on exercise capacity and gas exchange in patients with chronic heart failure. *Chest* 1996; 110: 985–991.

75. Keteyian SJ, Levine AB, Brawner CA et al. Exercise training in patients with heart failure. A randomised, controlled trial. *Ann Intern Med* 1996; 124: 1051–1057.

Specialist nurse intervention in chronic heart failure

Simon Stewart

10

The need for innovative strategies to optimize the management of older patients with chronic heart failure

There is little doubt that clinically proven therapeutics, such as angiotensin converting enzyme (ACE) inhibitors, spironolactone and beta-blockers have failed to have as great an impact on the dismal hospitalization and survival rates associated chronic heart failure as was first anticipated.[1] With the exception of one recent report, suggesting that survival following hospitalization for chronic heart failure had improved marginally,[2] most of the data (although these largely reflect the early years of ACE inhibition) are not encouraging. For example, chronic heart failure continues to be the leading cause of hospitalization among patients aged over 65 years in the USA[3,4] and recent studies of relatively unselected, but generally older, chronic heart failure patients report readmission rates of 35–65% in the 6 months following acute hospitalization.[5–8] The management of chronic heart failure costs at least 1–2% of all healthcare expenditure in Western countries;[9] the dominant component being the cost of hospitalization. The mortality in severe heart failure is 60% at

1 year.[10] In a recent population-based comparison of survival rates following a first hospitalization for heart failure with the most common forms of cancer specific to men and women, heart failure was shown to be associated with a 5-year survival rate of about 25% in both sexes, being second only to lung cancer in this regard.[11] Not only is chronic heart failure deadly but it is also associated with an extremely poor quality of life.[12]

The burden of chronic heart failure is likely to rise. Its prevalence increases with age, and society is ageing. Frailer patients, who would previously have died at a younger age, owing to less effective management of hypertension and ischaemic heart disease,[13] are surviving longer, even if a recent analysis of contemporary trends in hospitalization for chronic heart failure in Scotland would suggest that we are currently at the peak of this modern-day epidemic.[14]

This chapter identifies the major and mostly preventable factors that contribute to poorer health outcomes among older individuals with chronic heart failure. Appropriately designed programmes that incorporate the combination of specialist nurse leadership and home-based assessment and intervention have the potential to address many of these factors.

Factors that contribute to poor health outcomes in the chronically ill

The apparent inability of many individuals to gain the maximum clinical benefit from proven therapeutics is a multifactorial problem. This is not surprising, considering the complex interaction between the individual, the available treatments and the many components of the healthcare system in which they are managed. Suboptimal treatment is commonly the result of problems that hinder the interaction between the patient and the healthcare system. The degree to which this has an impact on an individual varies, depending on the stability and severity of disease state(s) and the relative safety of the therapeutic regimen. The consequences can therefore range from lack of symptomatic control to unplanned hospitalization and even premature death.

Unfortunately, older patients with chronic heart failure would benefit most from appropriate and consistent treatment, but are most vulnerable to those factors that cause suboptimal treatment. This is often compounded by their inability to tolerate even minor fluctuations in their condition, which in turn leaves them vulnerable to frequent and recurrent episodes of acute heart failure. *Figure 10.1* is a representation of the almost inevitable cycle of clinical improvement and deterioration in older chronic heart failure

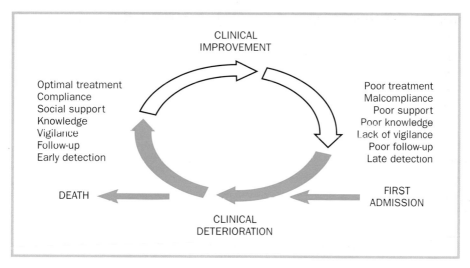

Figure 10.1

The characteristic cycle of clinical improvement and deterioration among hospitalized chronic heart failure patients

patients who require hospitalization for decompensated heart failure and who have therapeutic options limited to medical/palliative therapy.

Once a chronic heart failure patient has survived a first hospitalization for heart failure (especially if characterized by acute pulmonary oedema) they are at increased risk for further hospital admissions and, ultimately, premature death.[15-19] For many patients, the typically intensive treatment and clinical improvement associated with an acute hospitalization is followed by prolonged periods of clinical stability, minimal functional impairment and good quality of life (in comparison to similarly aged individuals), with only infrequent (and probably unavoidable) episodes of acute deterioration. There are a number of factors that help patients avoid episodes of deterioration (see left of *Figure 10.1*).

Conversely, a small proportion of patients (usually older, with more severe systolic dysfunction and concomitant chronic disease states) remain in a continual cycle of clinical improvement and deterioration. Disturbingly, there is recent evidence to suggest that the proportion of such patients is increasing.[14] Those factors responsible (listed on the right of *Figure 10.1*) are the complete opposite of those listed on the left. Such patients are much more likely to have a poorer quality of life, more severe functional impairment and recurrent (and costly) admissions to hospital. Furthermore, these patients are often admitted to hospital with multiple problems that confound their heart failure treatment (e.g. chronic airway limitation, diabetes and chronic renal failure).[20] It is this type of patient who has been identified as the high-cost user of healthcare resources.[21,22]

Pharmacological agents, such as ACE inhibitors and β-adrenoceptor blockers, stabilize the physiological consequences of heart failure and have proved to be partially effective.[10,23,24] However, even optimal drug combinations when closely monitored in the context of clinical trials (and their carefully selected cohorts) do not prevent negative outcomes. In addition, many preventable and inter-related factors may impact upon the health outcomes of chronic heart failure patients.

Inadequate or inappropriate pharmacotherapy

Although there are many guidelines for the diagnosis and management of chronic heart failure,[25,26] a large proportion of chronic heart failure patients continue to receive suboptimal treatment.[7,27–30] For example, ACE inhibitors are often either prescribed in subtherapeutic doses[30] or not prescribed at all. Patients

treated by specialist cardiologists are more likely to receive appropriate treatment[28,29] but most patients are treated by non-specialist physicians.

Non-adherence with prescribed treatment

Morbidity and perhaps mortality may be related to poor compliance and/or monitoring of prescribed pharmacotherapy. Studies examining the major determinants of poor adherence patterns among large patient populations consistently link non-adherence with the presence of chronic illness and a greater number of prescribed medications.[31–34] Almost 50% of chronically ill patients significantly deviate from prescribed pharmacotherapy.[32,35–37] Although it is more difficult to measure, there is little doubt that patients have similar problems adhering to fluid restriction and salt-reduced diets. Other frequently reported problems likely to impact upon adherence include difficulty in opening medication containers, hoarding and consuming old medications and regularly altering dosages (often without informing the treating physician). Physicians frequently overestimate the extent of their patients' adherence to prescribed treatment.[38] Not surprisingly, poor treatment adherence has been identified as a major precursor of readmissions among chronic heart failure patients.[39,40]

Adverse effects of prescribed treatment

Chronically ill patients are also at increased risk of being hospitalized because of adverse effects of their treatment. For example, approximately 2–15% of hospital admissions (depending on the criteria used) among chronically ill patients have been attributed to adverse effects of prescribed medication.[36,41–43] The benefits of drug therapy in the treatment of chronic heart failure has to be balanced against the increased risk of serious adverse effects in an elderly population.

Inadequate knowledge of chronic heart failure and prescribed treatment

Studies consistently demonstrate that patients have difficulty in recalling the potential adverse effects and/or special instructions pertaining to their prescribed medication.[31,32,44,45] This does not mean, however, that the other components of medication-related knowledge (such as the purpose, effect and intended effects of prescribed medication) are frequently known. Poor health-related knowledge is correlated with greater age, lower education levels and presence of a chronic illness;[32] the typical profile of many hospitalized chronic heart failure patients. How important is a good understanding of an illness and the treatment regimen? Greater knowledge does not necessarily lead to increased adherence to a regimen, and there is often a deficit between behavioural intention and action.[32,46,47] The relative efficacy of strategies designed to improve treatment adherence (e.g. reminder cards and pre-packaged doses) compared to those that aim to improve medication-related knowledge (e.g. pre-discharge counselling) remains unknown. On a practical basis, however, it is important to recognize that poor medication management usually represents a multitude of factors, and that implementation of multifaceted strategies that address both adherence and knowledge deficits make more sense than implementing one-dimensional strategies.

Inadequate follow-up and suboptimal use of available healthcare

Both the extent of follow-up care and the ability or willingness of patients to access such care have been identified as important determinants of health outcomes among the chronically ill.[48–50] Theoretically, providing greater follow-up care in order to increase the frequency of detecting and treating clinically unstable patients at subsequent risk of hospitalization is an attractive proposition. However, it would appear that markedly increasing patient contact with physicians who have the power to admit patients to hospital can increase hospitalization rates.[51] This is most probably due to the combination of an increased likelihood of detecting usually benign fluctuations in the patient's status and a lowering of the normal threshold at which patients would be hospitalized.[52]

Early clinical deterioration

Whilst almost all hospitalized chronic heart failure patients receive intensive treatment and stabilization followed by incremental follow-up, a significant proportion will rebound into hospital within weeks of their discharge as a result of early clinical deterioration.[48,53–55] Although the factors associated with this early rebound phenomenon are poorly characterized, older and more fragile patients with other chronic conditions that confound treatment are most at risk.

Suboptimal psychosocial support

There is a close association between poorer socioeconomic status and poorer health outcomes.[48,53] A major component of this risk relates to lack of social support. Poverty can limit social contacts (even via telephone) as well as contribute to poor diet and low uptake of medication. Individuals with chronic heart failure are at particular risk of becoming depressed.[56] Such patients also lack the support systems that would normally increase the likelihood of detecting emerging problems as well as providing both emotional and practical support in managing their chronic illness.

The evidence for incorporating specialist nurse intervention in the management of chronic heart failure

Many strategies have been developed to address the factors discussed above and reduce the frequency of hospitalization among chronically ill patients. Such strategies often include attention to one or more of the following: incremental discharge planning, follow-up using a specialist outpatient clinic; and home-based follow-up. Despite the theoretical attractiveness of such treatment regimens, results of previously reported randomized controlled studies of this type have been conflicting, with favourable,[41,54,57,58] inconclusive[49,50,59–63] and even unfavourable[51] effects reported on frequency and duration of readmission to hospital.

To date there have been six properly powered, randomized controlled studies of specialist nurse interventions that have included high proportions of chronic heart failure patients reported in the literature. The results of two further studies, recently completed in Glasgow, UK[64] and Auckland, New Zealand are yet to be published in full but support the literature thus far. There is already convincing evidence of the beneficial effects of strategies that involve the combined use of specialist nurse leadership and home-based intervention.[65]

Negative or inconclusive randomized controlled studies

Perhaps unsurprisingly, considering the inherent publication bias towards the reporting of positive studies, there is only one reported negative study in the literature. This was a study of 1396 male veterans hospitalized with chronic obstructive pulmonary disease, diabetes or heart failure who were randomized to either usual care or increased access to primary care nurses and physicians.[51] The intervention group had a greater number of readmissions to hospital, but were more satisfied with their medical care during 6 months of follow-up. It may be that the increased healthcare utilization resulted from a combination of greater vigilance in detecting problems and the ability of those detecting such problems (the physicians) to admit patients—thereby lowering admission thresholds.[52] This so-called 'clinical cascade' represents an important caveat when considering the potential impact of this type of intervention. For example, while increased nursing contact with patients is likely to result in more clinical problems being detected, there is also the potential for increased hospitalization rates if a specialist nurse is empowered to admit patients to hospital.

There have been two inconclusive trials of specialist nurse intervention. The first of these was a controlled study of a comprehensive discharge planning protocol implemented by advanced practice nurses. It demonstrated short-term, but not sustained, reductions in readmissions and decreased costs of care for older hospitalized patients with a number of medical cardiac conditions (including heart failure).[50] The same group has examined the additive effect of home-based follow-up (a series of home visits by advanced practice nurses).[66] The intervention was associated with fewer hospital readmissions and days of associated hospitalization within 24 weeks, but only a small proportion of patients had chronic heart failure and there was a significant amount of loss to follow-up (approximately 30%).

A more recent study[67] undertaken by Jaarsma and colleagues,[67] examined the effects of a heart failure-specific, home-based, educational programme undertaken by a specialist heart failure nurse. This study examined whether a single-type intervention designed to increase chronic heart failure patients' self-care behaviour could reduce hospital readmissions. However, despite sufficient sample size and a trend towards reduced hospital use, cost-effective thresholds were not reached. For example, during 9 months of follow-up, 37% of intervention patients (n = 84) versus 50% of usual care patients (n = 95) had a hospital readmission ($p = 0.06$). Patients exposed to the study intervention also tended to have fewer cardiac related days of readmission than the usual group (427 versus 681 days; $p = 0.096$).

Positive randomized controlled trials

In the first (and most important) study of its kind, Rich and colleagues demonstrated that a nurse-led, multidisciplinary intervention (involving a component of home visits) had beneficial effects on rates of hospital readmission, quality of life and cost of care within 90 days of discharge among high-risk chronic heart failure patients.[55] The intervention consisted of comprehensive education of the patient and family, a prescribed diet, social service consultation and planning for an early discharge, optimization of pharmacotherapy and intensive home- and clinic-based follow-up with frequent telephone contact. At 90 days, survival without readmission was achieved in 91 of 142 (64%) intervention patients compared to 75 of 140 (54%) control patients ($p = 0.09$). There were 94 versus 53 readmissions in the control and intervention groups, respectively ($p = 0.02$). Of the total readmissions 78 (53%) were for heart failure, and there was a disproportionate reduction (56%) of these types of readmission in the intervention group (24 versus 54; $p = 0.04$). Fewer intervention group patients had more than one readmission (9 versus 23; $p = 0.01$). These results were associated with significantly better quality of life and reduced health costs among intervention patients.

In Sweden, Cline and colleagues also demonstrated the benefits of a clinic-based follow-up of a lower-risk cohort of patients with chronic heart failure.[68] A total of 206 older patients hospitalized with heart failure were randomized to the study intervention or to usual care. The special intervention included an education programme for patients and their families, concentrating on treatment. Frequent and easily accessible patient-initiated follow-up was provided as a nurse-run, hospital-based clinic and telephone contact. During 12 months of follow-up, time to first readmission was a third longer in the intervention group (106 versus 141 days; $p < 0.05$). The intervention was also associated with a strong trend towards fewer hospital admissions, fewer days of hospitalization and lower cost of care during study follow-up.

In post-hoc analyses of a large-scale randomized controlled study of chronically ill patients with a mixture of cardiac and non-cardiac disease states,[41] we showed that a nurse-led, multidisciplinary, home-based intervention was most effective in chronic heart failure patients, in both the short[69] and the medium term.[70] We therefore prospectively examined the effects of a more heart failure-specific form of nurse-led, home-based intervention.[58] Chronic heart failure patients discharged to home after acute hospitalization were randomized to usual care (n = 100) or to the study intervention (n = 100). The intervention primarily consisted of a home visit at 7–14 days after discharge by a cardiac nurse to identify and address issues likely to result in unplanned hospitalization. During 6 months of follow-up, the primary end-point of unplanned readmission plus out-of-hospital death occurred more frequently in the usual care group (129 versus 77 primary events; $p = 0.02$). More intervention patients remained event-free (38 versus 51; $p = 0.04$), had fewer unplanned readmissions (68 versus 118; $p = 0.03$) and associated days of hospitalization (460 versus 1173; $p = 0.02$). Hospital-based costs for the intervention group tended to be lower than for the usual care group ($A 490 300 versus $A 922 600; $p = 0.16$). The mean cost of the intervention was $A 350 per patient, whilst other community-based costs were similar for both groups. Heart failure specific ($p = 0.04$) and general quality of life scores ($p = 0.01$) at 3 months were most improved among those patients assigned to the study intervention.

Blue et al, from Glasgow, found that home-based nurse intervention reduced the risk of death or hospitalization for heart failure from 53% in the usual core group to 37% ($p = 0.033$).[64]

Non-randomized studies

The positive results of the randomized studies described above are consistent with those of other non-randomized studies of similar strategies targeting older, hospitalized chronic heart failure patients. For example, Kornowski and colleagues reported that an intensive home-based intervention by physicians was associated with reduced hospitalization rates and quality of life in such patients.[71] West and colleagues reported that an intensive physician-supervised, nurse-mediated, home-based system for heart failure management (the MULTIFIT programme) was associated with improved functional status and exercise capacity and reduced hospitalization rates among both previously hospitalized and clinic-managed chronic heart failure patients.[72] Shah and colleagues have also reported the preliminary results of a study examining a nurse-led electronic monitoring programme, incorporating a strategy to facilitate patient self-monitoring with weekly reminder calls by nurses. The intervention reduced subsequent hospitalization among a small cohort (n = 27) of both older and middle-aged chronic heart failure patients.[73]

What are the key components of nurse intervention?

These results provide strong evidence that the implementation of programmes that combine specialist nurse leadership and home-based intervention have the greatest potential. The benefits of such programmes are summarized in *Table 10.1*. All the successful programmes of this type incorporate a multifaceted approach and use a specialist nurse as a cost-effective means for accurately identifying areas

Table 10.1
Potential benefits of specialist nurse-led home-based intervention

Preventable factor	Ideal outcome	Benefits of specialist nurse-led intervention
Non-prescription of proven therapeutic agents Prescription of subtherapeutic doses	Prescription patterns consistent with the current guidelines Titration of doses to therapeutic levels	Using strict protocols, properly trained and accredited nurses can initiate appropriate pharmacotherapy and titrate doses accordingly. Regular nurse monitoring (preferably in the home) may overcome the reluctance of many physicians to initiate new therapy or titrate doses upwards (for example, in the first stages of initiating a β-blocker because of anticipated clinical instability)
Poor adherence rates Increased risk of adverse effects of prescribed treatment	Optimal adherence to treatment Reduced incidence of adverse effects	Programmes incorporating specialist nurses and home-based intervention have been shown to improve treatment compliance and to limit medication-related admissions to hospital. By applying a multifaceted approach to the 'multitude of sins' often associated with medication management, it is difficult to pinpoint which components are most effective. However, the most important component is the ability to accurately assess the patient's needs in their own home
Early clinical deterioration	Prompt detection of deterioration resulting in incremental community-based treatment rather than costly readmission to hospital	By performing a comprehensive physical assessment and obtaining a careful history as part of a home visit in the immediate post-discharge period, there is a good chance that a specialist nurse will detect early clinical deterioration requiring immediate attention. As above, this may require adjustment of pharmacotherapy and/or addressing the issue of non-adherence. It will also prompt a change in the nature and frequency of the healthcare provided, as the nurse (and treating physicians) will have a better idea of the patient's therapeutic needs
Inadequate long-term follow-up Suboptimal use of available resources	Prompt detection of deterioration and provision of multidisciplinary services that consistently meet the patient's particular needs Patients and carers encouraged to participate in the day-to-day management of their chronic heart failure	Nurse-specialist intervention, especially when targeted towards high risk chronic heart failure patients, is a cost-effective means to provide more intensive and effective long-term follow-up of such patients. Ideally, the specialist nurse should be in a position to assess the patient's individual needs and make rapid referrals for incremental assessment and care (e.g. dietitian, pharmacist and social work). If patients (and family) are able to meet the nurse during hospitalization and then subsequently in their home, it is more likely that a good working relationship will be established. Furthermore, if the patient receives constructive and practical help to manage their condition in the process, they are more likely to access healthcare (or nurse) when problems arise
Suboptimal knowledge of chronic heart failure and its treatment	Optimal knowledge of the pathophysiological consequences of chronic heart failure Patients exhibit the ability to recognize when intended therapeutic outcomes are not being met	During hospitalization, older, chronic heart failure patients often suffer from the combination of physiological and psychological stress in addition to being passive participants in the management of their care. They are unlikely to remember the details of any in-hospital counselling. Conversely, the home, when the patient has probably re-established some normalcy and self-sufficiency, is the ideal location for educational support, especially if it encompasses the practical problem-solving of issues facing the patient and their family/carers. Educational strategies should also target the patient's family/carers and concentrate upon encouraging them to understand chronic heart failure and its treatment as well as promoting vigilance and prompt intervention for clinical deterioration
Poor psychosocial support	Patients receive the type of support that will make them feel more secure and cared for	The many chronic heart failure patients who move from the intensive care and attention in the hospital to the emptiness of home will naturally feel neglected. Furthermore, clinic visits to doctors are usually brief. More prolonged home or clinic visits with specialist nurses offers not only direct clinical benefits but also the opportunity to make the patient feel better cared for. Even though this type of benefit is difficult to measure, it is probably one of the most important components of such programmes

of suboptimal treatment and for providing a focal point for co-ordinating a multidisciplinary response to the needs of the patient.

A number of important issues need to be clarified in relation to achieving maximal cost-benefits. The most important issues relate to the optimal timing, intensity and duration of the intervention. For example, Rich's group in the USA used an intensive programme that lasted 3 months after hospitalization.[54] We in Australia used a less intensive (and potentially more cost-effective) programme[58,69,70] and yet both were associated with significantly fewer readmissions. Furthermore, Cline's group in Sweden implemented visits to nurse-led clinics for up to 8 months after discharge and offered consultations with a cardiologist at 1 and 4 months.[68] It may be possible to eliminate the non-productive, or least effective, components of programmes and still retain the beneficial effects, but the programmes need to be adapted to suit the particular characteristics of the patients being targeted (e.g. high- versus low-risk) and the strengths and weaknesses of the healthcare system in which they are managed, which will vary from one country to another. Regardless of differences in the intensity and duration of these programmes, however, there are a number of components that appear to be essential to their success:

- Use of highly trained cardiovascular nurses with appropriate qualifications and training to enable them to become semi-autonomous. Regular monitoring of their operational performance and effectiveness should be undertaken. That prospective appointees should have the appropriate interpersonal skills to establish good working relationships with their patients is just as important as ensuring that they have good clinical skills.

- Ensuring that nurses have the authority to initiate and/or titrate pharmacotherapy according to agreed protocols or, alternatively, have a defined pathway to ensure that this occurs rapidly following assessment of the patient's needs.

- Implementation of multifaceted strategies to address the complex problems that influence compliance, and encourage the patient/family to become more active in their own management.

- Implementation of multifaceted (e.g. verbal, written and visual) educational strategies designed to improve the patient's understanding of their condition and treatment but also that of their family/carer.

- Comprehensive liaison and consultation with other important members of the healthcare team (e.g. cardiologist, primary care physician, pharmacist, dietitian, social worker and community nurse) to provide a consistent and co-ordinated approach to the patient's management. Ideally, the nurse should be able to operate semi-independently by using the extended authority of the patient's cardiologist or specialist in order to expedite any remedial action required.

- Implementation of at least one prolonged visit to the patient's home (preferably in the 1–2-week period following discharge) to assess comprehensively and accurately how well the patient is coping in their own environment and to optimize treatment thereafter.

- Establishment of ongoing follow-up. This may take the form of further home visits, telephone calls, specialist-nurse clinics or a combination of all three.

Conclusions

We can do more for patients with chronic heart failure, especially older, hospitalized patients who face the prospect of recurrent episodes of acute clinical deterioration and frequent readmissions. The key to promoting better health outcomes is to address the problems that promote clinical instability. Programmes that incorporate the combination of specialist-nurse leadership and home-based intervention reduce hospital admissions, improve quality of life and reduce costs. Subject to fine tuning of the optimal nature, timing and duration of these programmes, they should be widely implemented and their efficacy tested among other patient groups with chronic heart failure (e.g. outpatient

clinic populations), in addition to patients with other chronic cardiac problems (e.g. those with atrial fibrillation).

References

1. McMurray J, McDonagh T, Morrison CE, Dargie HJ. Trends in hospitalization for heart failure in Scotland 1980–1990. *Eur Heart J* 1993; **14**: 1158–1162.

2. MacIntyre K, Capewell S, Stewart S et al. Evidence of improving prognosis in heart failure: trends in case-fatality in 66,547 patients hospitalised between 1986 and 1995. *Circulation* 2000; **102**: 1126–1131.

3. Hennen J, Krumholz HM, Radford MJ. Twenty most frequent DRG groups among Medicare inpatients age 65 or older in Connecticut hospitals, fiscal years 1991, 1992, and 1993. *Conn Med* 1995; **59**: 11–15.

4. Haldeman GA, Croft JB, Giles WH, Rashidee A. Hospitalization of patients with heart failure: national hospital discharge survey 1985–1995. *Am Heart J* 1999; **137**: 352–360.

5. Lowe J, Candlish P, Henry D et al. Management and outcomes of congestive heart failure: a prospective study of hospitalised patients. *Med J Aust* 1998; **168**: 115–118.

6. Krumholz HM, Parent EM, Tu N et al. Readmission after hospitalization for congestive heart failure among medicare beneficiaries. *Arch Intern Med* 1997; **157**: 99–104.

7. Reis SE, Holubkov R, Edmundowicz D et al. Treatment of patients admitted to the hospital with congestive heart failure: specialty-related disparities in practice patterns and outcomes. *J Am Coll Cardiol* 1997; **30**: 733–738.

8. Burns RB, McCarthy EP, Moskowitz MA et al. Outcomes for older men and women with congestive heart failure. *J Am Geriatr Soc* 1997; **45**: 276–280.

9. McMurray J, Davie A. The pharmacoeconomics of ACE inhibitors in chronic heart failure. *PharmacoEcon* 1996; **9**: 188–197.

10. The CONSENSUS Trial Study Group. Effects of enalapril on mortality in severe congestive heart failure: results of the Cooperative North Scandinavian Enalapril Survival Study. *N Engl J Med* 1987; **316**: 1429–1435.

11. Stewart S, MacIntyre K, Hole DJ et al. More malignant than cancer? Five-year survival following a first admission for heart failure in Scotland. *J Am Coll Cardiol* 2000; **35**: 551A.

12. Stewart AL, Greenfield S, Hays RD et al. Functional status and well-being of patients with chronic conditions—results from the medical outcomes study. *J Am Med Assoc* 1989; **262**: 907–913.

13. Ghali J, Cooper R, Ford E. Trends in hospitalization rates for heart failure in the United States, 1973–1986. *Arch Intern Med* 1990; **150**: 769–773.

14. Stewart S, MacIntyre K, MacLeod M et al. Trends in hospitalisation for heart failure in Scotland: an epidemic that has reached its peak? *Eur Heart J* 2000; in press.

15. Andersson B, Waagstein F. Spectrum and outcome of congestive heart failure in a hospitalized population. *Am Heart J* 1993; **126**: 632–640.

16. Cowburn P, Cleland J, Coats A, Komajda M. Risk stratification in chronic heart failure. *Eur Heart J* 1998; **19**: 696–710.

17. Hanyu N, Nauman D, Hershberger R. Managed care and outcomes of hospitalization among elderly patients with congestive heart failure. *Arch Intern Med* 1998; **158**: 1231–1236.

18. Wolinsky F, Smith D, Stump T et al. The sequelae of hospitalization for congestive heart failure among older adults. *J Am Geriatr Soc* 1997; **45**: 558–563.

19. Jaagosild P, Dawson N, Thomas C et al. Outcomes of acute exacerbation of severe congestive heart failure. *Arch Intern Med* 1998; **158**: 1081–1089.

20. Brown A, Cleland J. Influence of concomitant disease on patterns of hospitalization in patients with heart failure discharged from Scottish hospitals in 1995. *Eur Heart J* 1998; **19**: 1063–1069.

21. Zook CJ, Moore FD. High-cost users of medical care. *N Engl J Med* 1980; **302**: 996–1002.

22. McMurray J, Hart W, Rhodes G. An evaluation of the cost of heart failure to the National Health Service in the UK. *Br J Med Econ* 1993; **6**: 99–110.

23. The SOLVD Investigators. Effect of enalapril on survival in patients with reduced left ventricular ejection fractions and congestive heart failure. *N Engl J Med* 1991; **325**: 293–302.

24. MERIT Investigators. Effect of metoprolol CR/XL in chronic heart failure: Metoprolol CR/XL Randomised Intervention Trial in Congestive Heart Failure (Merit-HF). *Lancet* 1999; **353**: 2001–2007.

25. European Society of Cardiology Working Group on Heart Failure. Guidelines for the diagnosis of heart failure. *Eur Heart J* 1997; **16**: 741–751.

26. European Society of Cardiology Working

Group on Heart Failure. The treatment of heart failure. *Eur Heart J* 1997; **18**: 736–753.

27. Smith N, Psaty B, Pitt B et al. Temporal patterns in the medical treatment of congestive heart failure with angiotensin-converting enzyme inhibitors in older adults, 1989 through 1995. *Arch Intern Med* 1998; **158**: 1081–1098.

28. Stafford RS, Saglam D, Blumenthal D. National patterns of angiotensin-converting enzyme inhibitor use in congestive heart failure. *Arch Intern Med* 1997; **157**: 2460–2464.

29. Edep ME, Shah NB, Tateo IM, Massie BM. Difference between primary care physicians and cardiologists in management of congestive heart failure: relation to practice guidelines. *J Am Coll Cardiol* 1997; **30**: 518–526.

30. Luzier A, Forrest A, Adelman M et al. Impact of angiotensin-converting enzyme inhibitor underdosing on rehospitalization rates in congestive heart failure. *Am J Cardiol* 1998; **82**: 465–469.

31. Lowe CJ, Raynor DK, Courtney EA et al. Effects of self medication programme on knowledge of drugs and compliance with treatment in elderly patients. *Br Med J* 1995; **310**: 1229–1231.

32. Stewart S, Pearson S. Uncovering a multitude of sins: medication management in the home post acute hospitalisation among the chronically ill. *Aust NZ Med J* 1999; **29**: 220–227.

33. Stewart S, Davey M, Desanctis M et al. Home medication management: a study of patient post-hospitalisation. *Aust Pharmacist* 1995; **14**: 472–476.

34. Nikolaus T, Kruse W, Bach M et al. Elderly patients' problems with medication. An in-

hospital and follow-up study. *Eur J Clin Pharmacol* 1996; **49**: 255–259.

35. Eraker SA, Kirscht JP, Becker MH. Understanding and improving patient compliance. *Ann Intern Med* 1984; **100**: 258–268.

36. Rudd P, Ramesh J, Bryant-Kosling C, Guerrero D. Gaps in cardiovascular medication taking: the tip of the iceberg. *J Gen Intern Med* 1993; **8**: 659–666.

37. Blenkiron P. The elderly and their medication: understanding and compliance in a family practice. *Postgrad Med J* 1996; **72**: 671–676.

38. Donovan J, Blake D. Patient non-compliance: deviance or reasoned decision-making? *Soc Sci Med* 1992; **34**: 507–513.

39. Vinson JM, Rich MW, Sperry JC et al. Early readmission of elderly patients with congestive heart failure. *J Am Geriatr Soc* 1990; **38**: 1290–1295.

40. Gooding J, Jette AM. Hospital readmissions among the elderly. *J Am Geriatr Soc* 1985; **33**: 595–601.

41. Stewart S, Pearson S, Luke CG, Horowitz JD. Effects of a home based intervention on unplanned readmissions and out-of-hospital deaths. *J Am Geriatr Soc* 1998; **46**: 174–180.

42. Hewitt J. Drug-related unplanned readmissions to hospital. *Aust J Hosp Pharm* 1995; **25**: 400–403.

43. Col N, Fanale JE, Kronholm P. The role of medication noncompliance and adverse drug reactions in hospitalizations of the elderly. *Arch Intern Med* 1990; **150**: 841–845.

44. Furlong S. Do programmes of medicine self-administration enhance patient knowledge, compliance and satisfaction? *J Adv Nurs* 1996; **23**: 1254–1262.

45. Veggeland T, Fagerheim KU, Ritland T et al. [Do patients know enough about their medication? A questionnaire among cardiac patients discharged from 5 Norwegian hospitals]. *Tidsskrift Norske Laegeforening* 1993; **113**: 3013–3016.

46. McMahon T, Clark C, Bailie G. Who provides patients with drug information? *Br Med J* 1987; **294**: 355–356.

47. Conrad P. The meaning of medications: another look at compliance. *Soc Sci Med* 1985; **20**: 29–37.

48. Graham H, Livesley B. Can readmissions to a geriatric medical unit be prevented? *Lancet* 1983; **1**: 404–406.

49. Fitzgerald JF, Smith DM, Martin DK et al. A case manager intervention to reduce readmissions. *Arch Intern Med* 1994; **154**: 1721–1729.

50. Naylor M, Brooten D, Jones R et al. Comprehensive discharge planning for the hospitalized elderly. *Ann Intern Med* 1994; **120**: 999–1006.

51. Weinberger M, Oddone EZ, Henderson WG. Does increased access to primary care reduce hospital readmissions? *N Engl J Med* 1996; **334**: 1441–1447.

52. Mold JW, Stein HF. The cascade effect in the clinical care of patients. *N Engl J Med* 1986: 512–514.

53. Williams IE, Fitton F. Factors affecting early unplanned readmission of elderly patients to hospital. *Br Med J* 1988; **297**: 784–787.

54. Rich MW, Vinson JM, Sperry JC et al. Prevention of readmission in elderly patients with congestive heart failure: results of a prospective, randomized pilot study. *J Gen Intern Med* 1993; **8**: 585–590.

55. Rich MW, Beckham V, Wittenberg C et al. A multidisciplinary intervention to prevent the readmission of elderly patients with congestive heart failure. *N Engl J Med* 1995; **333**: 1190–1195.

56. Koenig HG. Depression in hospitalized older patients with congestive heart failure. *Gen Hosp Psych* 1998; **20**: 29–43.

57. Townsend J, Piper M, Frank AO et al. Reduction in hospital readmission stay of elderly patients by a community based hospital discharge scheme: a randomised controlled trial. *Br Med J* 1988; **297**: 544–547.

58. Stewart S, Marley JE, Horowitz JD. Effects of a multidisciplinary, home-based intervention on unplanned readmissions and survival among patients with chronic congestive heart failure: a randomised controlled study. *Lancet* 1999; **354**: 1077–1083.

59. Smith DM, Weinberger M, Katz BP, Moore PS. Post discharge care and readmissions. *Med Care* 1988; **26**: 699–708.

60. Rubin CD, Sizemore MT, Loftis PA et al. The effect of geriatric evaluation and management on Medicare reimbursement in a large public hospital: a randomized clinical trial. *J Am Geriatr Soc* 1992; **40**: 989–995.

61. Hansen FR, Spedtsberg K, Schroll M. Geriatric follow-up by home visits after discharge from hospital: a randomized controlled trial. *Age Ageing* 1992; **21**: 445–450.

62. Siu AL, Kravitz RL, Keeler E et al. Postdischarge geriatric assessment of hospitalized frail elderly patients. *Arch Intern Med* 1996; **156**: 76–81.

63. Weinberger M, Smith DM, Katz BP, Moore PS. The cost-effectiveness of intensive postdischarge care. *Med Care* 1988; **26**: 1092–1102.

64. Blue L, Strong E, Davie AP et al. Improving long-term outcome with specialist nurse intervention in heart failure: a randomised trial. *Eur Heart J* 2000; **21** (Abst. Suppl): 151.

65. McMurray J, Stewart S. Nurse-led, multidisciplinary intervention in chronic heart failure [Editorial]. *Heart* 1998; **80**: 430–431.

66. Naylor MD, Brooten D, Cambell R et al. Comprehensive discharge planning and home follow-up of hospitalized elders: a randomized clinical trial. *J Am Med Assoc* 1999; **281**: 613–620.

67. Jaarsma T, Halfens R, Huijer Abu-Saad H et al. Effects of education and support on self-care and resource utilization in patients with heart failure. *Eur Heart J* 1999; **20**: 673–682.

68. Cline C, Israelsson B, Willenheimer R et al. A cost effective management programme for heart failure reduces hospitalisation. *Heart* 1998; **80**: 442–446.

69. Stewart S, Pearson S, Horowitz JD. Effects of a home-based intervention among patients with chronic congestive heart failure. *Arch Intern Med* 1998; **158**: 1067–1072.

70. Stewart S, Vandenbroek A, Pearson S, Horowitz J. Prolonged beneficial effects of a home-based intervention on unplanned readmissions and mortality among congestive heart failure patients. *Arch Intern Med* 1999; **159**: 257–261.

71. Kornowski R, Zeeli D, Averbuch M et al. Intensive home-care surveillance prevents hospitalization and improves morbidity rates among elderly patients with severe congestive heart failure. *Am Heart J* 1995; **129**: 162–166.

72. West J, Miller N, Parker K et al. A comprehensive management system for heart failure improves clinical outcomes and reduces medical resource utilization. *Am J Cardiol* 1997; **79**: 58–63.

73. Shah NB, Der E, Ruggerio C et al. Prevention of hospitalizations for heart failure with an interactive home monitoring program. *Am Heart J* 1998; **135**: 373–378.

The patient with intractable heart failure: a practical guide to management

David R Murdoch

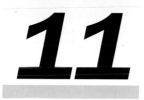

The morbidity and mortality of chronic heart failure due to left ventricular systolic dysfunction (LVSD) remains high despite recent advances in treatment. This is particularly so for patients with advanced symptoms. For example, in the CONSENSUS study, although mortality was substantially and significantly reduced by treatment with the angiotensin converting enzyme (ACE) inhibitor enalapril, mortality in these patients with severe symptoms was still 26% at 6 months.[1] In addition, most patients with chronic heart failure have significant lifestyle limitations and their quality of life fares poorly when compared with that in other chronic conditions.[2] A significant minority of such patients remain incapacitated with intractable oedema, breathlessness or exercise intolerance despite standard modern therapy consisting of a loop diuretic, ACE inhibitor, spironolactone, beta-blocker and digoxin. This chapter will address the management of these 'resistant' patients.

Confirmation of the diagnosis

The clinical diagnosis of both symptomatic and asymptomatic LVSD is difficult and unreliable, owing to a high prevalence in the community of conditions that may mimic the signs and symptoms of heart failure such as chronic obstructive airways disease, obesity with exercise intolerance, orthostatic oedema and varicose insufficiency.[3] In a community study of all patients diagnosed as having definite heart failure only 50% subsequently had significant impairment of left ventricular systolic function confirmed at echocardiography.[4] Thus, in all cases an objective measure of left ventricular function is essential to the diagnosis of heart failure, especially for those thought to have intractable symptoms resistant to standard therapy (see Chapter 3).[5,6] Other routine investigations should search for alternative or contributory causes and include a chest X-ray, assessment of renal and hepatic function, assessment of haemoglobin, and in some cases pulmonary function testing and plasma ferritin assay.

Optimization of standard therapy

The approach to patients considered to have 'intractable' heart failure is shown in *Figure 11.1*.

Non-pharmacological treatment

Few patients with chronic heat failure have any knowledge of their disease. Consequently, simple measures, such as fluid and salt restriction, which improve symptoms and reduce diuretic requirements, are rarely adopted (see Chapter 9).

One of the main reasons for death in heart failure is recurrent ischaemic events, as evidenced by the major post-myocardial infarction ACE inhibitor studies.[7–9] Therefore, cessation of smoking is essential and general nutrition should be improved, while all patients should adopt sensible alcohol consumption, and those with alcoholic cardiomyopathy should abstain completely.

A sensible approach to regular exercise should also be adopted by patients within the limits of their symptoms.

Reduction or withdrawal of unnecessary or harmful drugs

In general, unnecessary drugs should be withdrawn. Specifically, non-steroidal anti-inflammatory drugs (NSAIDs) promote salt and water retention, reduce the effectiveness of ACE inhibitors and exacerbate renal dysfunction, especially with concomitant ACE inhibitor therapy. Their use in heart failure should be strongly discouraged.[10] In most patients with degenerative arthritis, substitution of NSAIDs with paracetamol or simple compound analgesia is usually equally effective. Similarly, many patients with ischaemic heart disease are taking low-dose aspirin therapy for secondary preventive effects. Remarkably, recent evidence suggests that this too may reduce the effectiveness of

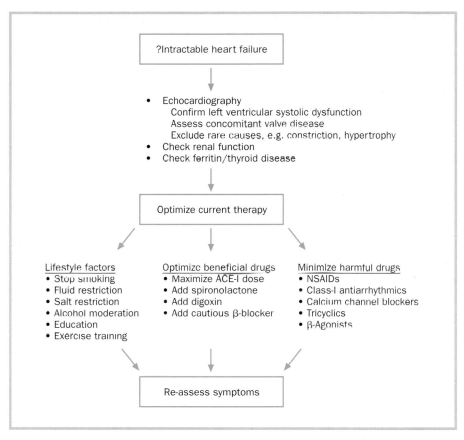

Figure 11.1
Initial approach to the management of the patient considered to have intractable heart failure.

ACE inhibitors[11–13] and that the dose should be reduced to the minimum effective dose, probably 75 mg daily.[14,15] There is no evidence that aspirin should be given to patients with idiopathic dilated cardiomyopathy. Consideration should be given to substitution of aspirin with warfarin, especially when concomitant paroxysmal or sustained atrial fibrillation or left ventricular thrombus formation makes this clearly advantageous. Whether routine warfarinization confers any benefit over aspirin in patients with heart failure is controversial but is being addressed by the ongoing WATCH study. Theophylline, β-agonist bronchodilators and tricyclic antidepressants may also exacerbate heart failure and should be avoided wherever possible. Class I antiarrhythmics have been shown to have an adverse effect on mortality and should be discontinued. Similarly, calcium channel blockers, with the possible exception of amlodipine, should be discontinued unless essential.[16]

Optimization of therapy associated with improved symptoms and prognosis

ACE inhibitors

The considerable benefits on mortality and morbidity conferred by the use of ACE inhibitors in patients with all grades of heart failure and asymptomatic left ventricular dysfunction are now undisputed.[1,17-19] It is of primary importance, therefore, that all patients with chronic heart failure receive treatment with adequate doses of a proven agent. While there seems little to choose between the different agents available, it seems prudent to use a drug that has been proven in clinical trials and where 'target' doses have been established (*Table 11.1*). This is especially so in patients with severe symptoms who have the most to gain from treatment, in

absolute terms, when compared with those with milder symptoms.

Following the publication of the ELITE II study,[20] it has become clear that angiotensin II, type 1 receptor blockers (AT_1) are not superior to ACE inhibitors in chronic heart failure. ACE inhibitors must, therefore, remain the first choice in chronic heart failure except where cough makes ACE inhibitors intolerable, where AT_1 blockers are a reasonable substitute.

Spironolactone

Following publication of the RALES study,[25] spironolactone has become essential therapy for patients with moderate or severe symptoms of chronic heart failure (NYHA III or IV). This randomized, double-blind, placebo-controlled, study of 1663 patients showed impressive morbidity and mortality effects of adding a conventionally very low dose of spironolactone (initially 25 mg, maximum of 50 mg) to standard therapy including an ACE inhibitor. The trial stopped prematurely, owing to a reduction in mortality of 30% with active treatment. Of greater importance is the finding that spironolactone therapy was associated with significant improvements in the symptoms of heart failure, as evidenced by improvements in NYHA class, and that patients were 35% less likely to be admitted to hospital for chronic heart failure decompensation. The main

Table 11.1
Choice of ACE inhibitor: recommended doses of commonly used agents

Trial	SOLVD[16]	SAVE[17]	AIRE*[21]	Smile*[22]	GISSI-3*[23]	ISIS-4*[24]
Drug	Enalapril	Captopril	Ramipril	Zofenopril	Lisinopril	Captopril
Initial dose	2.5 mg	6.25 mg	2.5 mg	7.5 mg	5 mg	6.25 mg
Titration	2.5 mg BD	25 mg TDS in Hospital	2.5 mg BD for 2 days	7.5 mg after 12 hours	5 mg after 24 hours	12.5 mg after 2 hours
	5 mg BD	50 mg TDS thereafter	5 mg BD thereafter	dose doubled	10 mg after 48 hours	25 mg 10–12 hours later
	10 mg BD				10 mg OD thereafter	50 mg BD thereafter
Target dose	10 mg BD	50 mg TDS	5 mg BD	30 mg BD	10 mg OD	50 mg BD

* Post infarction trials

exclusions were serum levels of potassium of >5.0 mmol/l and creatinine of >221 μmol/l, and side-effects were limited to gynaecomastia in 10% of men. The mean increase in serum potassium was only 0.30 mmol/l and significant hyperkalaemia (>6.0 mmol/l) was found in only 2% of those on spironolactone, as compared with 1% of placebo-treated patients.

Although the mean dose of spironolactone in RALES was 26 mg daily, the protocol allowed for an increase to 50 mg daily after 8 weeks if the patient showed evidence of progression of their symptoms. The fact that this occurred more frequently in the placebo-treated patients, where the mean placebo dose was 31 mg, and was not limited by

hyperkalaemia in those on spironolactone, is a further indicator of the efficacy of the drug in these patients with severe symptoms. It seems prudent that, for the patients with intractable symptoms, who are eligible to receive spironolactone, the target dose should be 50 mg daily. Caution is necessary. There are anecdotal reports of life-threatening hyperkalaemia in patients treated with spironolactone. Potassium should be checked within a few days of starting therapy.

β-Blockade

Three large placebo-controlled randomized trials have recently been published examining the effect of β-blockade on mortality and morbidity in addition to standard therapy in chronic heart failure—The US Carvedilol Program (carvedilol),[26] CIBIS-II (bisoprolol)[27] and MERIT-HF (metoprolol CR/XL).[28] These trials have mainly recruited patients with mild or moderate symptoms (NYHA II-III), and the proportion of class IV patients has been small, and the benefit uncertain. A pooled analysis of all NYHA IV patients in these trials (n = 622) does, however, suggest that such treatment may be beneficial. Mortality in placebo-treated patients was 22.7% (71/213) compared with 17.5% (53/309) in those treated with β-blockade. Of greater importance is the COPERNICUS study, which was recently prematurely terminated because of substantial benefit in carvedilol-treated patients. This trial recruited patients with severe symptoms and there was a 35% reduction in mortality with carvedilol.

Initial doses should be small (e.g. 1.25 mg bisoprolol OD, 3.125 mg carvedilol BD or 15.5 mg CR/XL metoprolol OD), as there is a risk of precipitating decompensation, especially in those with severe symptoms.

Physical training

It is now well know that the central haemodynamic function of the heart at rest correlates poorly with the functional capacity of the patient. One of the mechanisms involved in reduced physical tolerance is peripheral dysfunction, including reduction in muscle mass, decreased muscle blood flow and reduced skeletal muscle oxygen utilization.[29] There is now considerable evidence that physical training increases leg blood flow and muscle mass, has beneficial skeletal muscle metabolic effects, reduces sympathetic tone and increases vagal tone. In those with moderate or severe heart failure, there are associated increases in endurance, muscle strength, quality of life and functional capacity.[30] A tailored training programme should be considered routine care in all heart failure patients. Unfortunately, local availability of this specialist service is currently very limited. For further discussion, see Chapter 9.

Identification of the primary problem

Intractable oedema or pulmonary congestion

There can be little doubt that, from a patient's perspective, the most effective treatment for heart failure is a loop diuretic. Diuretics improve all symptoms of the syndrome including oedema, breathlessness and exercise intolerance, although, naturally, there are very few placebo-controlled studies of their efficacy.[31,32]

Patients with severe gravitational oedema and/or pulmonary oedema are best admitted to hospital for initiation of treatment (*Figure 11.2*). Usually a diuresis can be established with the intravenous administration of a loop diuretic, e.g. frusemide 50–100 mg twice daily. Although exercise restriction may be detrimental in heart failure, a period of bed rest for 24–48 hours is still of value for those with severe oedema. Where possible, urinary catheterization is best restricted to those with acute severe pulmonary oedema, as it adversely affects movement and quality of life, in addition to the inherent mechanical and infective complications. Careful fluid balance combined with daily weighing, clinical assessment, and regular analysis of urea and electrolytes is a suitable substitute for most patients.

For those in whom intermittent intravenous diuretic therapy fails to cause sufficient diuresis, the intravenous infusion of a loop agent, e.g. frusemide 10 mg/hour, is more effective (dose for dose) than intermittent therapy and may help to initiate a diuresis for those with diuretic resistance.[33,34] This can be titrated to 20 mg and 40 mg/hour in the most resistant patients. Unfortunately, diuretic infusions usually require urinary catheterization, as nocturia may be intolerable.

When oedema has been controlled by intravenous diuretics, oral therapy can be substituted. There is little to choose between frusemide and bumetanide in this setting;

however, bumetanide has more consistent bioavailability, has less variable absorption after food and may reduce plasma potassium to a lesser degree than frusemide.[35–37] For patients with severe oedema requiring prolonged intravenous therapy, a suitable oral dose is 2 mg twice daily of bumetanide or 80 mg twice daily of frusemide, depending on renal function. Only if this fails to maintain a stable body weight should additional or combination diuretic therapy be considered.

For the few patients who fail to diurese with an intravenous infusion of loop diuretic of adequate dose according to renal function, the addition of a thiazide diuretic is usually required. Although metolazone is commonly used, there is no evidence that it is any more efficacious than a standard thiazide diuretic. In the only published comparative trial, bendrofluazide was as effective as metolazone for combination therapy.[38] For either agent, 5 mg daily for 3 days appears as efficacious as longer therapy for initiating a diuresis. Metolazone is slowly absorbed and has a long elimination half-life (2 days). This may account for the observed delay in clinical effect. Combination therapy has the potential to cause major biochemical abnormalities and its use must be carefully monitored with respect to both renal function and the rate of fluid loss. Intermittent or continuous metolazone (or bendrofluazide) outpatient therapy can be very helpful in the management of patients with recurrent

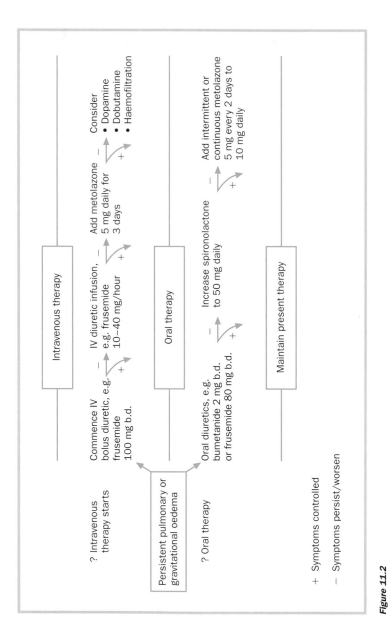

Figure 11.2
Diuretic and concomitant therapy in severe pulmonary or gravitational oedema.

oedema who would otherwise require recurrent, prolonged hospital admissions. A suitable maintenance dose for outpatient therapy would be 5 mg of either agent every second day initially, increasing cautiously towards a maximum dose of 10 mg daily if essential.

Chronic inotrope therapy has been uniformly disappointing in chronic heart failure. In some acute situations, its use is unavoidable, particularly where hypotension complicates severe unresponsive oedema. The evidence for benefit from pulsed therapy with dobutamine is controversial, but there may be some role for low-dose therapy in severely disabled patients.[39] Low-dose dopamine has theoretical advantages, as selective dopaminergic stimulation causes renal arterial dilatation at relatively low doses. Unfortunately, recent studies of the oral, selective DA-1 and DA-2 receptor agonist, ibopamine, were terminated prematurely because of a significant excess of deaths in the active treatment group.[40] Indeed, of the oral agents subjected to randomized clinical trial, all have demonstrated an adverse mortality effect.[41,42]

Peripheral perfusion and urinary flow are of greater importance than blood pressure per se. In severe hypotension, dobutamine (5 μg/kg per minute and titrated upwards to achieve adequate vital organ perfusion) can be used in the absence of prominent tachycardia. Low-dose dopamine (2.5 μg/kg per minute)

can improve urine output but does not improve renal function. Higher doses are rarely helpful as α-adrenergic effects exacerbate peripheral vasoconstriction. In clinical practice, a combination of both of these is often used. Recent unpublished data suggest that the calcium sensitizer levosimendan may increase survival compared to both placebo and dobutamine. In general it seems wise to restrict the use of inotropic drugs to those in whom symptoms are considered more important than mortality.

There is substantial evidence for the use of intravenous vasodilators, particularly nitrates, in the treatment of acute severe left heart failure with pulmonary oedema.[43,44] Nitrates reduce right heart pressures and pulmonary capillary wedge pressure when given by repeated bolus or continuous infusion, although their continuous use in chronic heart failure is limited by tolerance. Interestingly, evidence suggests that concomitant hydralazine,[45] or perhaps ACE inhibitors,[46] may reduce the development of nitrate tolerance. Where blood pressure is well maintained, however, intravenous nitrate therapy can prove a useful addition to standard therapy when given at low dosage (1 mg/hour) for 24–48 hours. It may be particularly useful in those with concomitant myocardial ischaemia. Sodium nitroprusside may also be useful in this situation.

Exertional dyspnoea and exercise intolerance

While oedema as a result of fluid retention can usually be controlled by careful titration of diuretic agents, exercise intolerance often persists and remains difficult to treat with pharmacological therapy (*Figure 11.3*).

High dose ACE inhibition

There is now some evidence to support a widely held belief amongst heart failure specialists that higher doses of ACE inhibitors may be more effective than lower doses. In the ATLAS study of 3164 patients with stable NYHA II-IV chronic heart failure over 36 months,[47] 'high-dose' lisinopril (32.5 to 35 mg daily) compared with 'low-dose' lisinopril (2.5 to 5 mg daily) was associated with an additional 8% (not significant) risk reduction in the primary end-point of all-cause mortality and 12% ($p = 0.002$) risk reduction in the combined secondary end-point 'a priori' of all-cause mortality plus all-cause hospitalizations. Furthermore, the incidence of symptomatic hypotension or renal dysfunction was similar between the groups. In another smaller study, high-dose ACE inhibition (10 mg imidapril) was associated with improvements in exercise time and physical working capacity when compared with lower-dose regimes (2.5 or 5 mg) over a 3-month period.[48]

The NETWORK study of three dosage regimes of enalapril (2.5, 5 or 10 mg all twice daily), showed no dose–response relationship in 1532 patients with chronic heart failure.[49] However, NETWORK was considerably smaller than ATLAS and compared three rather similar dosage regimes over a shorter 6-month follow-up period. In addition, most patients in NETWORK had mild symptoms (65% NYHA II), with a low-incidence Q wave infarction on the electrocardiogram (ECG) (24%).

Patients with resistant symptoms should, therefore, receive the highest tolerated dose of ACE inhibitor, e.g. 40 mg daily of enalapril (20 mg twice daily) or lisinopril. In this setting modest hypotension should generally be tolerated in the absence of evidence of vital organ hypoperfusion. Other vasodilators, such as calcium antagonists (which have not been associated with favourable prognostic benefits) should be stopped unless there is some other indication, such as angina.

Optimise digoxin dose

While the recently published DIG study showed no mortality advantage with the addition of digoxin to standard ACE inhibitor and diuretic therapy in patients with heart failure who remained in sinus rhythm, there was an impressive reduction in hospital admissions for cardiac de-compensation (60 prevented per 1000 years of treatment).[50]

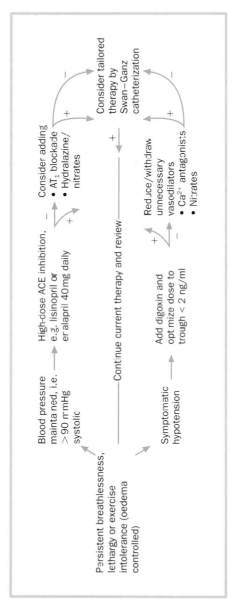

Figure 11.3
Options for pharmacological or tailored therapy in the patient with persistent severe breathlessness or exercise tolerance.

Furthermore, there were 40 fewer hospitalizations of any type per 1000 patient years of treatment. Subgroup analysis suggested that patients with more severe heart failure had the greatest absolute and relative benefit from digoxin therapy.[50] The dose of digoxin used in this study was calculated from a nomogram with a median daily dose of 250 µg. Mean achieved plasma digoxin level was 0.86 ng/ml (no attempt was made to optimize therapy according to plasma level). Many patients were thus undertreated. The question as to whether adjusting the dose according to plasma levels will provide additional clinical benefits is likely to remain unanswered.

The two studies of digoxin withdrawal, the PROVED[51] and RADIANCE[52] trials, provide some support for a more tailored approach. Here substitution of placebo in place of optimized digoxin therapy (target plasma level 0.7–2.0 ng/ml) was associated with worsening heart failure and increasing admissions to hospital. Therefore, in the presence of intractable symptoms it is possible that a higher plasma concentration may give additional benefit; titration up to a trough of 2 ng/ml is suggested in the absence of symptoms of toxicity.

Combination hydralazine and nitrates

Prior to the introduction of ACE inhibitors, high-dose hydralazine (target dose 300 mg/day) and oral nitrate therapy (ISDN target dose 160 mg/day) were shown to provide significant morbidity and mortality benefits in chronic heart failure,[53] although the combination was subsequently shown to be less effective than ACE inhibitors alone.[54] As a result, the use of the hydralazine/nitrate combination has fallen out of favour. For the significant minority of patients who remain intolerant to ACE inhibitors, particularly if because of renal dysfunction, the hydralazine/nitrate combination is an alternative. For those with severe symptoms, combination vasodilator therapy (hydralazine/nitrates and ACE inhibitors) can be considered, particularly with persistent hypertension, which should be aggressively controlled.

Combination ACE-I and AT$_1$ receptor blockade

Plasma concentrations of angiotensin II and aldosterone, however, remain elevated in patients with chronic heart failure despite treatment with an ACE inhibitor.[55,56] This persistent activation of the RAAS may be explained, at least in part, by the existence of non-ACE pathways that convert angiotensin I to angiotensin II.[57,58] ACE inhibitors, however, have another potentially important action in addition to RAAS blockade: the inhibition of bradykinin breakdown. This action does seem to contribute to the pharmacological effects of ACE inhibitors in humans.[59] Combination therapy with an ACE inhibitor and angiotensin II receptor antagonist may, therefore, offer the best therapeutic approach to blockade of the RAAS in patients with severe chronic heart failure.

The acute and chronic haemodynamic and neurohormonal actions of adding losartan,[60,61] valsartan[62] and candesartan[63] to an ACE inhibitor have been reported. These data suggest that combination therapy attenuates progressive left ventricular dilatation, and causes more profound inhibition of the RAAS, when compared with either an ACE or AT_1 blocker alone. We have found little significant incremental benefit in haemodynamic studies of the addition of an AT_1 receptor antagonist to ACE inhibitor therapy in patients with mild to moderate controlled chronic heart failure on optimal ACE inhibition, although combination therapy considerably reduced blood pressure.[64] Trials such as CHARM and Val-HeFt will assess the morbidity and mortality effects of combination therapy.[65,66] The Val-HeFt study has recently been presented and provides some evidence for this approach (American Heart Association, New Orleans, November 2000). Here the addition of high dose valsartan (40 mg BD increasing to 160 mg BD) was not associated with a significant reduction in the primary endpoint of mortality (19.7% vs. 19.4%) but significantly reduced the co-primary combined endpoint of mortality and

morbidity by 13% (28.8% vs. 32.1%, $p = 0.009$), mainly due to a reduction in the number of hospitalizations for worsening heart failure (27% RRR, $p < 0.00001$). Pending further data, it now seems reasonable to consider adding valsartan in those with severe symptoms, particularly when plagued by recurrent hospitalizations.

Other treatment considerations

Treatment of concomitant angina

As much as a third of patients with heart failure have angina.[16] Revascularization should always be considered in such patients as, while their operative risk is higher than that in patients with normal left ventricular function, paradoxically they may enjoy a greater survival benefit.[67] However, in patients with severe heart failure, the operative risk may be considered unacceptably high. Important exceptions are patients whose heart failure is predominantly due to ischaemic mitral regurgitation or obstructive valvular disease. Percutaneous revascularization (PTCA) remains an alternative therapy for those with isolated stenoses but, as yet, there is no evidence that this method of revascularization improves the prognosis in heart failure.

Medical treatment of angina in the presence of severe heart failure can be difficult. While nitrate therapy and the long-acting dihydropyridine calcium antagonist amlodipine appears safe in chronic heart failure,[68] the use of diltiazem[69] and short-acting nifedipine[70] have been associated with adverse mortality effects and should be avoided. ACE inhibitors themselves can have unpredictable effects on anginal frequency in those with ischaemic cardiomyopathy, perhaps by reducing coronary blood flow across critical stenoses.[71] The most effective treatment is likely to be the gradual introduction of β-blockers.

Invasive monitoring and 'tailored' vasodilatation

A number of reports have suggested that 'tailored vasodilatation', aimed at normalizing pulmonary artery wedge pressure and systemic vascular resistance, results in a better clinical outcome than empirical treatment with ACE inhibitors.[72–74] There are reported associated, substantial and long-term haemodynamic improvements with such an approach and reduced requirements for transplantation. Nevertheless, for the majority of patients who exhibit evidence of volume overload with good central and peripheral perfusion, empirical treatment with clinical monitoring until congestion is relieved is all that is required. In many patients with severe heart failure, however, ACE inhibitor therapy may be limited by symptomatic hypotension or the persistence of intractable exertional symptoms despite apparently optimal therapy. It can

often be difficult in such circumstances to accurately determine fluid status clinically; invasive haemodynamic monitoring by means of Swan–Ganz catheterization can provide important information regarding profiles of filling pressures and cardiac output with which to guide therapy. This may be particularly valuable where, for example, the presence of chronic pulmonary disease or renal failure further complicates the accurate clinical assessment of fluid balance.

Ultrafiltration and haemodialysis

There is often a close relationship between cardiac and renal function in advanced heart failure. Consequently, the treatment of heart failure in those with significant renal dysfunction is considerably more troublesome. Conversely, the presence of intrinsic renal disease may precipitate overt heart failure in those with only mild or moderate LVSD who may otherwise be asymptomatic. It is occasionally necessary to consider either temporary dialysis (haemo- or peritoneal) or ultrafiltration to help initiate a diuresis in those with predominant cardiac dysfunction or to initiate renal replacement therapy in those with a predominance of renal failure.

Pacemakers: conventional and multisite pacing

Pacemakers are not infrequently required in

the treatment of heart failure, most commonly to correct an inappropriately low heart rate on account of sick sinus syndrome. Intermittent or chronic high-degree atrioventricular (AV) block also constitutes a class I indication for pacing. It is particularly important to maintain normal AV conduction by dual chamber pacing whenever possible, as this has been shown to reduce morbidity and prolong survival in chronic heart failure patients.[75,76] In some cases the use of rate-responsive and mode-switching generators should be considered to maximize exercise capacity, and minimize the effects of paroxysmal atrial fibrillation, respectively.

There have been several recent advances in pacing modalities in heart failure, which have been made possible by advances in pacing technology. Initial trials of sequential AV pacing with a short AV delay using 'standard' dual-chamber pacemakers for patients who remain in sinus rhythm have been disappointing, with no improvement in pump function or clinical status over time.[77] Generators are, however, now commercially available which are capable of pacing both right and left ventricular myocardium concomitantly ('biventricular' or three-chamber pacemakers). This may allow a more co-ordinated ventricular contraction and minimize the adverse effects of intraventricular conduction defects that are common in patients with advanced heart failure.[78] The technical limitation to this

technique was previously the need for thoracotomy to allow for placement of the left ventricular lead. This is, however, now possible transvenously by placement of a pacing electrode through the coronary sinus in a cardinal vein. Biventricular pacing (see *Figure 11.4*) consistently reduces ECG QRS duration and in some studies has been associated with significant improvements in exercise tolerance,[79] and left ventricular ejection fraction.[80] It is likely to be of most benefit to those with significant intraventricular conduction abnormalities and QRS widening, especially if combined with

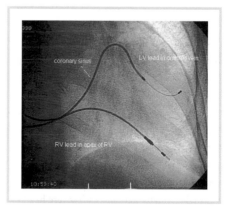

Figure 11.4
Biventricular pacing. Plain radiograph, right anterior oblique view. The right ventricular lead has been placed in the apex of the right ventricle using active fixation. The left ventricular lead is position in a vein draining the left ventricle via the coronary sinus

AV conduction disease. Prediction of long-term improvement may be related to the reduction in QRS duration.[81] At least one long-term study is underway to evaluate the functional and symptomatic improvement with biventricular pacing in chronic heart failure (VIGOR CHF).

Surgical options

Conventional revascularization procedures

Ischaemic heart disease is the predominant cause of chronic heart failure in the Western world. In an unknown, but perhaps considerable, proportion of patients, reversible rather than permanent ischaemic dysfunction may predominate or contribute to ventricular dysfunction. Chronically hypoperfused myocytes can remain viable but 'hibernating' and may recover when revascularized. Such a mechanism might be responsible for the improved prognosis demonstrated in the CASS study in patients with severe coronary disease and left ventricular systolic impairment.[67] The prospect of revascularization in chronic heart failure, especially in those with severe intractable symptoms, is limited by the considerable operative mortality rate. Nevertheless, in patients with severe ischaemia, who demonstrate viability of tissue by thallium scanning or contractile reserve by stress

echocardiography, this should be considered. There is currently no evidence that angioplasty improves the outcome of these patients, although anginal symptoms may be improved.

Aneurysmectomy, Batista and other remodelling operations

Resection of an aneurysmal segment of the left ventricle, usually combined with bypass grafting, has an established place in the management of suitably selected patients with heart failure. Recently, a novel approach has been described for patients with dilated cardiomyopathy where the geometry of the left ventricle is returned towards normal by resection of a segment of left ventricular wall.[81] This reduces the end-systolic dimension and associated functional mitral regurgitation. This and similar techniques are currently under evaluation.

Left ventricular assist devices and 'artificial hearts'

A number of left ventricular assist devices are now commercially available, e.g. Heartmate and Novacor in both the USA and UK. They are currently undergoing evaluation mainly in those with severe symptoms who await transplantation. All augment systolic and diastolic function by means of an implantable electric pump operated by an external battery pack. Most attach to the left ventricular apex and aorta and 'bypass' the left ventricle, and some provide pulsatile flow. There are now several case reports of these devices causing sufficient improvement in left ventricular function to be subsequently withdrawn. They may, therefore, be particularly valuable in those with reversible left ventricular systolic dysfunction as a result of, for example, myocarditis.

Education and non-pharmacological intervention

Education is crucial to the successful management of the patient with severe heart failure and is best delivered by both counselling and provision of written material in booklet format.[82,83] This should encompass all aspects of the management of the heart failure syndrome and is often best delivered by a specialist nurse and/or the multidisciplinary approach offered by specialized heart failure clinics (see Chapter 10).[84]

Special situations
Atrial fibrillation

Atrial fibrillation is associated with a worse prognosis compared with sinus rhythm in heart failure.[85] Atrial transport may contribute up to 30% of cardiac output in severe chronic heart failure and atrial fibrillation may lead to worsening of symptoms, owing to loss of atrial transport. Warfarin is important in atrial

fibrillation or paroxysmal atrial fibrillation associated with heart failure, as the risk of thromboembolism is high.

Whenever possible, attempts should be made to restore sinus rhythm. Unfortunately, although cardioversion may provide significant symptom relief, long-term maintenance is difficult as left atrial dilatation due to high left atrial pressure or significant mitral regurgitation is common. Nevertheless, unless the rhythm has been particularly long-standing or the left atrium is particularly dilated, at least one attempt at DC cardioversion should be made. Pretreatment with amiodarone is safe and increases the likely success of cardioversion and the duration of sinus rhythm once it has been achieved.[86] For some patients, the benefits of long-term amiodarone to maintain sinus rhythm outweigh the risks of side-effects with long-term treatment.

For those in whom sinus rhythm cannot be achieved, control of ventricular rate is important. Digoxin is traditionally used, but rate control with exercise often remains poor with digoxin alone. β-Blocker therapy gives better control of rate. In all cases sick-sinus syndrome must be excluded as, in this case, symptoms may be improved by a permanent pacemaker.

Obstructive valvular disease

The presence of obstructive valvular disease, particularly aortic stenosis, makes the treatment of heart failure difficult. Rarely, patients with mitral stenosis may present with 'heart failure'. Aortic stenosis is increasingly common as a result of the increasing frequency of degenerative valvular disease in the elderly. In addition to its effects on left ventricular function and cardiac output, aortic stenosis complicates the treatment of heart failure. Management is difficult and depends mainly on the severity of stenosis and the extent of left ventricular dysfunction or concomitant coronary artery disease. Where the stenosis is severe (gradient >60 mmHg) surgical valve replacement is the treatment of choice if the associated surgical risk is acceptable. It should also be appreciated that, in the presence of significant LVSD, Doppler echocardiography often underestimates the severity of stenosis. Where valve replacement is not possible, and LVSD is severe, there is evidence from small studies that cautious ACE inhibitor treatment may benefit some patients.[87,88] Balloon aortic valvuloplasty has largely been abandoned, except as a bridge to surgery, because of poor long-term results.

Mitral and aortic regurgitation

A degree of mitral regurgitation frequently accompanies heart failure, even where the mitral valve is structurally normal, due to stretching of the mitral valve annulus. In severe left ventricular dilatation such mitral regurgitation may become significant. It is important, though difficult, to establish in such cases whether the mitral regurgitation is truly functional and whether it is secondary rather than aetiological. While mitral valve replacement may benefit the latter, it will be of little value as sole therapy in the former. The symptoms of heart failure in moderate or severe mitral regurgitation are likely to be improved by conventional medical therapy including ACE inhibitors and β-blockers.

Patients with chronic aortic regurgitation who develop symptoms of heart failure are best stabilized by medical therapy before surgical intervention. The risk of aortic valve replacement here is dependent upon the severity of left ventricular dysfunction and in particular the left ventricular end-systolic dimension.

Renal artery stenosis

Patients with heart failure frequently have advanced disseminated atherosclerotic vascular disease, including significant renovascular disease. The prevalence of significant renal artery stenosis (>50%) is about 20% in patients with angiographically proven coronary disease.[89] This has a number of implications for the patient with heart failure:

1. Renovascular disease exacerbates heart failure as a result of further activation of the RAAS.

2. The resulting decline in renal function makes effective diuretic treatment difficult.
3. Significant renovascular disease complicates the use of ACE inhibitors.

In most patients with heart failure the pathology of renal artery stenosis is that of aortic atherosclerosis involving the origin of the renal artery rather than renal arterial disease per se. Suboptimal dilatation and unacceptable rates of re-stenosis accompanied previous attempts at angioplasty. More recently, however, the technical success and long-term results have been improved by elective stenting to include the origin of the renal artery. Stenting may help the treatment of patients with intractable symptoms with improvements in renal function allowing reduction of diuretic requirements and the introduction of ACE inhibitor therapy. Renal artery stenosis should be suspected in patients with heart failure and poor renal function or decline in renal function following the introduction of ACE inhibitors. These patients should be considered for renal angiography with a view to renal arterial stenting as appropriate.

Transplantation

Heart transplantation is now an accepted mode of treatment for end-stage heart failure and it should be considered at an early stage in those with 'intractable' symptoms. In selected patients, heart transplantation significantly increases survival, exercise capacity and ability to return to work. Recent studies suggest a 5-year survival of 70–80% for those on modern immunosuppressive therapy. The availability of heart transplantation is largely dependent upon organ supply and the demand greatly exceeds supply. In addition, there are many important contraindications to transplantation, including severe renal or hepatic impairment, alcohol abuse or continued smoking, fixed elevated pulmonary vascular resistance, significant systemic disease and advanced age. It is, therefore, most suitable for younger patients with uncontrollable symptoms but without additional significant disease. Besides shortage of donor hearts, the main problem of transplantation is rejection of the allograft or complications of immunosuppression, e.g. renal failure or accelerated atherosclerosis including transplant coronary artery disease.

The truly intractable patient

Fortunately, relatively few patients with chronic heart failure have either continuous rest symptoms or continually progressive symptoms despite optimal, individually tailored, medical treatment. Urgent heart transplantation is often considered, but many patients in this situation are elderly or are ineligible, owing to multisystem pathology. Here considerations of symptomatic relief and reducing the duration and frequency of hospital admission often take priority over mortality reduction. In such severely affected patients hypotension is common and it is often necessary to reduce ACE inhibitors, vasodilators and β-blockers for periods of time in preference to intensive diuretic therapy and intermittent recourse to inotropes. Invasive monitoring by Swan–Ganz catheterization can be useful and occasionally produces surprising results. Multidisciplinary home monitoring by community physicians and nurse specialists is invaluable to help identify decompensation at an early stage and either organize urgent elective admission to a specialist centre or institute additional treatment, such as short term oral thiazide therapy, to help keep patients at home.

Future treatment modalities

There have been tremendous advances in heart failure management over the past two decades, and the future of heart failure research has never looked brighter. There is likely to be further progress made by refinement of strategies to inhibit inappropriate neurohormonal activation with ACE inhibition and angiotensin receptor antagonists, and the introduction of new classes of drugs. With the ever-increasing number of drugs now used routinely in all grades of chronic heart failure, including diuretics, ACE inhibitors, β-blockers,

spironolactone, digoxin and AT_1 receptor blockade, identification of patient subgroups who benefit most from individual agents is also likely to become more important with time.

Potential future treatment modalities in heart failure are listed in *Table 11.2*. Two of these, which are already in clinical trials, deserve special attention.

Endothelin-1 (ET-1) is a potent pressor peptide synthesized in the vasculature and myocardium. Plasma concentrations of ET-1 are raised in chronic heart failure, correlate

Table 11.2
Potential future treatment modalities for heart failure

Endothelin receptor antagonism, e.g. bosentan
Anticytokine therapy, e.g. anti-TNFα (etanercept)
Neutral endopeptidase inhibitors, e.g. ecadotril, candoxatril (enhances plasma levels and the effects of ANP and BNP)
Combined NEP and ACE inhibition, e.g. omapatrilat, sampatrilat
Metabolic therapy, e.g. ʟ-carnitine
Combination ACE and AT_1 receptor blockade
Left ventricular assist devices and artificial hearts
Xenotransplantation

TNF, tumour necrosis factor; ANP and BNP, natriuretic peptides; NEP, neutral endopeptidase; ACE, angiotensin converting enzymes; AT_1, angiotensin II type 1 receptor

with the symptomatic and haemodynamic severity, and predict prognosis. Its cardiovascular actions are thought to be mediated primarily by endothelin-A (ET_A) and endothelin-B (ET_B) receptors, stimulation of the former generally causing vasoconstriction, the later vasodilatation. The functional significance of ET_B receptors in chronic heart failure is currently not clear and whether a selective ET_A receptor antagonist will be preferable to a non-selective ET_A/ET_B antagonist remains to be determined. The first of this new class of drugs, bosentan (a combined ET_A/ET_B antagonist) is now undergoing clinical trials. Provisional studies suggest that bosentan has favourable haemodynamic effects in chronic heart failure reducing right and left heart pressures and increasing cardiac index,[90] effects that are sustained with short-term oral therapy.[91]

Plasma concentrations of inflammatory cytokines are increased in patients with heart failure and correlate with the severity of symptoms. Research has centred on the potential aetiological role of tumour necrosis factor-α (TNFα) in severe heart failure and particularly in patients who develop the wasting syndrome, cardiac cachexia.[92] Such inflammatory cytokines can depress myocardial function, stimulate myocyte apoptosis and induce myocardial fibrosis. An entirely new avenue of treatment is now possible with the inhibition of such detrimental circulating cytokines. One approach is to use the soluble P75 TNF receptor (etanercept) that binds irreversibly with TNFα. Two large multicentre studies are currently underway with etanercept in severe chronic heart failure (RENAISSANCE and RECOVER). The oral xanthine derivative pentoxyfilline has anti-TNFα activity, and has already shown promising results in dilated cardiomyopathy in terms of improvements in symptoms and left ventricular ejection fraction.[93] It is, however, a complex drug with significant phosphodiesterase III inhibition which may have contributed to its clinical effects.

Conclusions

- Despite recent advances in treatment, a significant minority of patients with heart failure have intractable symptoms.
- Confirmation of the presence of left ventricular systolic dysfunction and identification of valvular abnormalities by echocardiography is mandatory in all patients with suspected heart failure, especially in those with intractable symptoms.
- A search for remediable contributory causes such as valvular disease and renal artery stenosis should always be considered.
- Fluid retention can normally be controlled by combination diuretic therapy, although recurrence is common and associated with frequent hospital admissions.

- The use of the highest tolerated dose of ACE inhibitors remains the cornerstone of management in these patients.

- The treatment of exercise intolerance remains problematic and is best by intensive vasodilator therapy and physical training. Invasive monitoring may be a useful guide to therapy in those whose symptoms persist despite apparently optimal fluid balance.

- The addition of digoxin has become established as standard therapy in those remaining symptomatic despite ACE inhibitors and diuretics. Optimization of dose according to plasma concentration may provide additional benefit in those with intractable symptoms.

- Recent evidence from randomized trials such as COPERNICUS suggests that β-blockade is of value even in those with severe symptoms (NYHA IV) if started cautiously with very low doses.

- Young patients with uncontrollable severe symptoms should be considered for transplantation at an early stage.

References

1. Swedberg K. Effects of enalapril on mortality in severe congestive heart-failure—results of the cooperative-north-scandinavian-enalapril-survival study (CONSENSUS). *N Engl J Med* 1987; **316**: 1429–1435.

2. Stewart AL, Greenfield S, Hays RD et al. Functional status and well-being of patients with chronic conditions—results from the medical outcomes study. *J Am Med Assoc* 1989; **262**: 907–913.

3. Remes J, Miettinen H, Reunanen A, Pyorala K. Validity of clinical diagnosis of heart failure in primary health care. *Eur Heart J* 1991; **12**: 315–321.

4. Wheeldon NM, MacDonald TM, Flucker CJ et al. Echocardiography in chronic heart failure in the community. *Q J Med* 1993; **86**: 17–23.

5. Davie AP, Francis CM, Love MP et al. Value of the electrocardiogram in identifying heart-failure due to left-ventricular systolic dysfunction. *Br Med J* 1996; **312**: 222.

6. Davie AP, Francis CM, Caruana L et al. Assessing diagnosis in heart failure: which features are any use? *Q J Med* 1997; **90**: 335–339.

7. Rutherford JD, Pfeffer MA, Moye LA et al. Effects of captopril on ischemic events after myocardial infarction. Results of the Survival and Ventricular Enlargement trial. SAVE Investigators. *Circulation* 1994; **90**: 1731–1738.

8. Yusuf S, Pepine CJ, Garces C et al. Effect of enalapril on myocardial infarction and unstable angina in patients with low ejection fractions. *Lancet* 1992; **340**: 1173–1178.

9. Hall AS, Murray GD, Ball SG. Follow-up study of patients randomly allocated ramipril or placebo for heart failure after acute myocardial infarction: AIRE Extension (AIREX) Study. *Lancet* 1997; **349**: 1493–1497.

10. Sturrock ND, Struthers AD. Non-steroidal anti-inflammatory drugs and angiotensin converting enzyme inhibitors: a commonly prescribed combination with variable effects on renal function. *Br J Clin Pharmacol* 1993; **35**: 343–348.

11. Cleland JG, Bulpitt CJ, Falk RH et al. Is aspirin safe for patients with heart failure? *Br Heart J* 1995; 74: 215–219.

12. Hall D, Zeitler H, Rudolph W. Counteraction of the vasodilator effects of enalapril by aspirin in severe heart failure. *J Am Coll Cardiol* 1992; 20: 1549–1555.

13. Nguyen KN, Aursnes I, Kjekshus J. Interaction between enalapril and aspirin on mortality after acute myocardial infarction: subgroup analysis of the cooperative new scandinavian enalapril survival study ii (CONSENSUS II). *Am J Cardiol* 1997; 79: 115–119.

14. Nyman I, Larsson H, Wallentin L. Prevention of serious cardiac events by low-dose aspirin in patients with silent-myocardial-ischemia. *Lancet* 1992; 340: 497–501.

15. Juulmoller S, Edvardsson N, Jahnmatz B et al. Double-blind trial of aspirin in primary prevention of myocardial-infarction in patients with stable chronic angina-pectoris. *Lancet* 1992; 340: 1421–1425.

16. Packer M, O'Connor CM, Ghali JK et al. Effect of amlodipine on morbidity and mortality in severe chronic heart failure (PRAISE). *N Engl J Med* 1996; 335: 1107–1114.

17. The SOLVD Investigators. Effect of enalapril on survival in patients with reduced left ventricular ejection fractions and congestive heart failure. *N Engl J Med* 1991; 325: 293–302.

18. Pfeffer MA, Braunwald E, Moye LA et al, for The SAVE Investigators. Effect of captopril on mortality and morbidity in patients with left ventricular dysfunction after myocardial infarction. Results of the survival and ventricular enlargement trial. *N Engl J Med* 1992; 327: 669–677.

19. Nicklas JM, Pitt B, Timmis G et al. Effect of enalapril on mortality and the development of heart-failure in asymptomatic patients with reduced left-ventricular ejection fractions. *N Engl J Med* 1992; 327: 685–691.

20. Pitt B, Poole-Wilson PA, Segal R et al. Effect of losartan compared with captopril on mortality in patients with symptomatic heart failure: randomised trial—the losartan heart failure survival study (ELITE-II). *Lancet* 2000; 355: 1582–1587.

21. The Acute Infarction Ramipril Efficacy (AIRE) Study Investigators. Effect of ramipril on mortality and morbidity of survivors of acute myocardial infarction with clinical evidence of heart failure. *Lancet* 1993; 342: 821–828.

22. Ambrosioni E, Borghi C, Magnani B. The effect of the angiotensin-converting-enzyme inhibitor zofenopril on mortality and morbidity after anterior myocardial infarction. The Survival of Myocardial Long-Term Evaluation (SMILE) Study Investigators. *N Engl J Med* 1995; 332. 80–85.

23. Gruppo Italiano per lo Studio della Sopravvivenza nell'infarto Miocardio. GISSI-3: effects of lisinopril and transdermal glyceryl trinitrate singly and together on a 6-week mortality and ventricular function after acute myocardial infarction. *Lancet* 1994; 343: 1115–1122.

24. ISIS-4 (Fourth International Study of Infarct Survival) Collaborative Group. ISIS-4: a randomised factorial trial assessing early oral captopril, oral mononitrate, and intravenous magnesium sulphate in 58,050 patients with suspected acute myocardial infarction. *Lancet* 345: 669–685.

25. Pitt B, Zannad F, Remme WJ et al, for the Randomised Aldactone Study Investigators (RALES). The effect of spironolactone on morbidity and mortality in patients with

severe heart failure. *N Engl J Med* 1999; **341:** 709–717.

26. Packer M, Bristow MR, Cohn JN, et al. The effect of carvedilol on morbidity and mortality in patients with chronic heart failure. U.S. Carvedilol Heart Failure Study Group. *N Engl J Med* 1996; **334:** 1349–1355.

27. The cardiac insufficiency bisoprolol study II (CIBIS-II): a randomised trial. *Lancet* 1999; **11:** 138–142.

28. Hjalmarson A, Goldstein S, Fagerberg B et al. Effect of metoprolol CR/XL in chronic heart failure: metoprolol CR/XL randomised intervention trial in congestive heart failure (MERIT-HF). *Lancet* 1999; **353:** 2001–2007.

29. Clarke A, Poole-Wilson P, Coats A. Exercise limitation in chronic heart failure: central role of the periphery. *J Am Coll Cardiol* 1996; **28:** 1092–1102.

30. Balardinelli R, Georgiou D, Scocco V et al. Low intensity exercise training in patients with chronic heart failure. *J Am Coll Cardiol* 1995; **26:** 975–982.

31. Patterson JH, Adams KF, Applefeld MM et al. Oral torsemide in patients with chronic congestive-heart-failure—effects on body-weight, edema, and electrolyte excretion. *Pharmacotherapy* 1994; **14:** 514–521.

32. Sherman LG, Liang CS, Baumgardner S et al. Piretanide, a potent diuretic with potassium-sparing properties, for the treatment of congestive-heart-failure. *Clin Pharmacol Ther* 1986; **40:** 587–594.

33. Dormans TP, van Meyel JJ, Gerlag PG et al. Diuretic efficacy of high dose furosemide in severe heart failure: bolus injection versus continuous infusion. *J Am Coll Cardiol* 1996; **28:** 376–382.

34. Lahav M, Regev A, Ra'anani P, Theodor E. Intermittent administration of furosemide vs continuous infusion preceded by a loading dose for congestive heart failure. *Chest* 1992; **102:** 725–731.

35. McCrindle JL, Li Kam Wa TC, Barron W, Prescott LF. Effect of food on the absorption of frusemide and bumetanide in man. *Br J Clin Pharmacol* 1996; **42:** 743–746.

36. Gabriel R, Baylor P. Comparison of the chronic effects of bendrofluazide, bumetanide and frusemide on plasma biochemical variables. *Postgrad Med J* 1981; **57:** 71–74.

37. Ramsay LE, McInnes GT, Hettiarachchi J et al. Bumetanide and frusemide: a comparison of dose–response curves in healthy men. *Br J Clin Pharmacol* 1978; **5:** 243–247.

38. Channer KS, Mclean KA, Lawsonmatthew P, Richardson M. Combination diuretic treatment in severe heart-failure—a randomized controlled trial. *Br Heart J* 1994; **71:** 146–150.

39. DICE Collaborative Group. Ambulatory intermittent 6-month low-dose dobutamine infusion in severe heart failure: DICE multicenter trial. *J Am Coll Cardiol* 1997; **29:** 17147 (abstract).

40. Hampton JR, VanVeldhuisen DJ, Kleber FX et al. Randomised study of effect of ibopamine on survival in patients with advanced severe heart failure. *Lancet* 1997; **349:** 971–977.

41. Packer M, Carver JR, Rodeheffer RJ et al. Effect of oral milrinone on mortality in severe chronic heart failure. The PROMISE Study Research Group. *N Engl J Med* 1991; **325:** 1468–1475.

42. Packer M, Rouleau J, Swedberg K et al. Effect of flosequinan on survival in chronic heart-failure—preliminary-results of the profile study. *Circulation* 1993; **88:** 301.

43. Northridge D. Frusemide or nitrates for acute heart failure? *Lancet* 1996; **347**: 667–668.

44. Cotter G, Metzkor E, Kaluski E et al. Randomised trial of high-dose isosorbide dinitrate plus low-dose furosemide versus high-dose furosemide plus low-dose isosorbide dinitrate in severe pulmonary oedema. *Lancet* 1998; **351**: 389–393.

45. Elkayam U, Canetti M, Wani OR et al. Hydralazine-induced prevention of nitrate tolerance: experimental and clinical evidence and potential mechanisms. *Am J Cardiol* 1998; **81**: A44–A48.

46. Munzel T, Bassenge E. Long-term angiotensin-converting enzyme inhibition with high-dose enalapril retards nitrate tolerance in large epicardial arteries and prevents rebound coronary vasoconstriction in vivo. *Circulation* 1996; **93**: 2052–2058.

47. Packer M, Poole-Wilson PA, Armstrong PW et al, on behalf of the ATLAS Study Group. Comparative effects of low and high doses of the angiotensin-converting enzyme inhibitor, lisinopril, on morbidity and mortality in chronic heart failure. *Circulation* 1999; **100**: 2312–2318.

48. Veldhuisen DJ, Genth-Zotz S, Brouwer J et al. High- versus low-dose ACE inhibition in chronic heart failure: a double-blind, placebo controlled study of imidapril. *J Am Coll Cardiol* 1998; **32**: 1811–1818.

49. Poole-Wilson P, Cleland J, Hubbard W et al. Clinical outcome with enalapril in symptomatic chronic heart failure; a dose comparison. *Eur Heart J* 1998; **19**: 481–489.

50. Perry G, Brown E, Thornton R et al. The effect of digoxin on mortality and morbidity in patients with heart failure. *N Engl J Med* 1997; **336**: 525–533.

51. Uretsky BF, Young JB, Shahidi FE et al. Randomized study assessing the effect of digoxin withdrawal in patients with mild-to-moderate chronic congestive-heart-failure—results of the PROVED trial. *J Am Coll Cardiol* 1993; **22**: 955–962.

52. Packer M, Gheorghiade M, Young JB et al. Withdrawal of digoxin from patients with chronic heart-failure treated with angiotensin-converting enzyme-inhibitors. *N Engl J Med* 1993; **329**: 1–7.

53. Cohn JN, Archibald DG, Ziesche S et al. Effect of vasodilator therapy on mortality in chronic congestive-heart-failure—results of a veterans-administration cooperative study (V-HeFT). *N Engl J Med* 1986; **314**: 1547–1552.

54. Cohn JN, Johnson G, Ziesche S et al. A comparison of enalapril with hydralazine–isosorbide dinitrate in the treatment of patients with chronic congestive heart failure (V-HeFT II). *N Engl J Med* 1991; **325**: 303–310.

55. Struthers AD. Aldosterone escape during ace-inhibitor therapy in chronic heart-failure. *Eur Heart J* 1995; **16**: 103–106.

56. Benedict CR, Francis GS, Shelton B et al. Effect of long-term enalapril therapy on neurohormones in patients with left-ventricular dysfunction. *Am J Cardiol* 1995; **75**: 1151–1157.

57. Voors AA, Pinto YM, Buikema H et al. Dual pathway for angiotensin II formation in human internal mammary arteries. *Br J Pharmacol* 1998; **125**: 1028–1032.

58. Akasu M, Urata H, Kinoshita A et al. Differences in tissue angiotensin II-forming pathways by species and organs in vitro. *Hypertension* 1998; **32**: 514–520.

59. Gainer JV, Morrow JD, Loveland A et al. Effect of bradykinin-receptor blockade on the

response to angiotensin-converting-enzyme inhibitor in normotensive and hypertensive subjects. *N Engl J Med* 1998; **339:** 1285–1292.

60. Hamroff G, Blaufarb I, Mancini D et al. Angiotensin II receptor blockade further reduces afterload safely in patients maximally treated with angiotensin-converting enzyme inhibitors for heart failure. *J Cardiovasc Pharmacol* 1997; **30:** 533–536.

61. Hamroff G, Katz SD, Mancini D et al. Addition of angiotensin II receptor blockade to maximal angiotensin-converting enzyme inhibition improves exercise capacity in patients with severe congestive heart failure. *Circulation* 1999; **99:** 990–992.

62. Baruch L, Anand I, Cohen IS et al. Augmented short- and long-term hemodynamic and hormonal effects of an angiotensin receptor blocker added to angiotensin converting enzyme inhibitor therapy in patients with heart failure. Vasodilator Heart Failure Trial (Val-HeFT) Study Group. *Circulation* 1999; **99:** 2658–2664.

63. McKelvie RS, Yusuf S, Pericak D et al. Comparison of candesartan, enalapril, and their combination in congestive heart failure—randomized evaluation of strategies for left ventricular dysfunction (RESOLVD) pilot study—the RESOLVD pilot study investigators. *Circulation* 1999; **100:** 1056–1064.

64. Murdoch DR, McDonagh TA, Morton JJ et al. Haemodynamic effects of the addition of eprosartan, a specific AT_1 receptor antagonist, to ACE inhibitor therapy in chronic heart failure. *Eur Heart J* 1998; **19:** 2214 (abstract).

65. Swedberg K, Pfeffer M, Granger C et al. Candesartan in Heart Failure—Assessment of Reduction in Mortality and Morbidity (CHARM): rationale and design. *J Cardiac Failure* 1999; **5:** 276–282.

66. Cohn JN, Tognoni G, Glazer RD et al. Rationale and design of the valsartan heart failure trial: a large multinational trial to assess the effects of valsartan, an angiotensin-receptor blocker, on morbidity and mortality in chronic congestive heart failure. *J Cardiac Failure* 1999; **5:** 155–160.

67. Alderman EL, Fisher LD, Litwin P et al. Results of coronary artery surgery in patients with poor left ventricular function (CASS). *Circulation* 1983; **68:** 785–795.

68. Packer M, O'Connor CM, Ghali JK et al. Effect of amlodipine on morbidity and mortality in severe chronic heart failure. Prospective Randomized Amlodipine Survival Evaluation Study Group (PRAISE). *N Engl J Med* 1996; **335:** 1107–1114.

69. Goldstein RE, Boccuzi SJ, Cruess D, Nattel S, the Adverse Experience Committee. The Multicentre Diltiazem Post Infarction Research Group. Diltiazem increases late onset congestive heart failure in post-infarction patients with early reduction in ejection fraction. *Circulation* 1991; **83:** 52–60.

70. Elkayam U, Amin J, Mehra A et al. A prospective, randomised, double-blind, cross-over study to compare the efficacy and safety of chronic nifedipine therapy to isosorbide dinitrate and their combination in the treatment of chronic congestive heart failure. *Circulation* 1990; **82:** 1954–1961.

71. Cleland JGF, Henderson E, McLenachan J et al. Effect of captopril, an angiotensin-converting enzyme inhibitor, in patients with angina pectoris and heart failure. *J Am Coll Cardiol* 1991; **17:** 733–739.

72. Fonarow GC, Chelimskyfallick C, Stevenson

LW et al. Effect of direct vasodilation with hydralazine versus angiotensin converting enzyme inhibition with captopril on mortality in advanced heart failure—the Hy-C trial. *J Am Coll Cardiol* 1992; **19**: 842–850.

73. Steimle AE, Stevenson LW, Chelimskyfallick C et al. Sustained hemodynamic efficacy of therapy tailored to reduce filling pressures in survivors with advanced heart failure. *Circulation* 1997; **96**: 1165–1172.

74. Stevenson LW, Dracup KA, Tillisch JH. Efficacy of medical therapy tailored for severe congestive heart-failure in patients transferred for urgent cardiac transplantation. *Am J Cardiol* 1989; **63**: 461–464.

75. Alpert MA, Curtis JJ, Sanfelippo JF et al. Comparative survival after permanent ventricular and dual chamber pacing for patients with chronic high degree atrioventricular-block with and without preexistent congestive-heart-failure. *J Am Coll Cardiol* 1986; **7**: 925–932.

76. Alpert MA, Curtis JJ, Sanfelippo JF et al. Comparative survival following permanent ventricular and dual-chamber pacing for patients with chronic symptomatic sinus node dysfunction with and without congestive-heart-failure. *Am Heart J* 1987; **113**: 958–965.

77. Gold MR, Feliciano Z, Gottlieb SS, Fisher ML. Dual-chamber pacing with short atrioventricular delay in congestive heart failure: a randomized study. *J Am Coll Cardiol* 1995; **26**: 967–973.

78. Kerwin WF, Botvinick EH, O'Connell JW et al. Ventricular contraction abnormalities in dilated cardiomyopathy: effect of biventricular pacing to correct interventricular dyssynchrony. *J Am Coll Cardiol* 2000; **35**: 1221–1227.

79. Leclercq C, Victor F, Alonso C et al. Comparative effects of permanent biventricular pacing for refractory heart failure in patients with stable sinus rhythm or chronic atrial fibrillation. *Am J Cardiol* 2000; **85**: 1154–1158.

80. Alonso C, Leclercq C, Victor F et al. Electrocardiographic predictive factors of long-term clinical improvement with multisite biventricular pacing in advanced heart failure. *Am J Cardiol* 1999; **84**: 1417–1421.

81. McCarthy M. Batista procedure proves its value in the USA. *Lancet* 1997; **349**: 855.

82. Kostis JB, Rosen RC, Cosgrove NM et al. Nonpharmacologic therapy improves functional and emotional status in congestive-heart-failure. *Chest* 1994; **106**: 996–1001.

83. Goodyer LI, Miskelly F, Milligan P. Does encouraging good compliance improve patients clinical condition in heart-failure? *Br J Clin Pract* 1995; **49**: 173–176.

84. Stewart S, Marley JE, Horowitz JD. Effects of a multidisciplinary, home-based intervention on unplanned readmissions and survival among patients with chronic congestive heart failure: a randomised controlled study. *Lancet* 1999; **354**: 1077–1083.

85. Middlekauff HR, Stevenson WG, Stevenson LW. Outcome for advanced heart failure patients with atrial fibrillation. *Cardiol Board Rev* 1992; **9**: 101–102.

86. Gosselink ATM, Crijns HJGM, VanGelder IC et al. Low-dose amiodarone for maintenance of sinus rhythm after cardioversion of atrial-fibrillation or flutter. *J Am Med Assoc* 1992; **267**: 3289–3293.

87. Martinez Sanchez C, Henne O, Arceo A et al. Hemodynamic effects of oral captopril in

patients with critical aortic stenosis. *Arch Inst Cardiol Mex* 1996; **66:** 322–330.

88. Grace AA, Brooks NH, Schofield PM. Beneficial effects of angiotensin converting enzyme inhibitors in severe symptomatic aortic stenosis. *Eur Heart J* 1991; **12:** 129 (abstract).

89. Jean WJ, AlBitar I, Zwicke DL et al. High-incidence of renal-artery stenosis in patients with coronary-artery disease. *Cathet Cardiovasc Diagn* 1994; **32:** 8–10.

90. Kiowski W, Sutsch G, Hunziker P et al. Evidence of endothelin-1 mediated vasoconstriction in severe chronic heart failure. *Lancet* 1995; **346:** 732–736.

91. Sutsch G, Bertel O, Kiowski W. Acute and short-term effects of the non-peptide endothelin-1 receptor antagonist bosentan in humans. *Cardiovasc Drugs Ther* 1997; **10:** 717–725.

92. McMurray J, Abdullah I, Dargie HJ, Shapiro D. Increased concentrations of tumour necrosis factor in 'cachectic' patients with severe chronic heart failure. *Br Heart J* 1991; **66:** 356–358.

93. Sliwa K, Skudicky D, Candy G et al. Randomised investigation of effects of pentoxifylline on left-ventricular performance in idiopathic dilated cardiomyopathy. *Lancet* 1998; **351:** 1091–1093.

Index